D0648499

CREATURE COMFORTS

CREATURE COMFORTS

The Adventures of a City Vet

Stephen Kritsick, D.V.M.
and
Patti Goldstein

Coward-McCann, Inc.
New York

Library of Congress Cataloging in Publication Data

Kritsick, Stephen.
  Creature comforts.

  1. Kritsick, Stephen.   2. Veterinarians—New
York (N.Y.)—Biography.   I. Goldstein, Patti.   II. Title.
SF613.K74A33   1983   636.089′092′4   [B]   82-22076
ISBN 0-698-11221-0

Printed in the United States of America

For my family.
S. K.

For Hug, Ollie and Kato with whom it all began—
and Wallis, who saw it through.

P. G.

CREATURE COMFORTS

Chapter 1

For at least eight hours every night, beginning at 5:00 P.M., the emergency treatment of most of the sick or injured animals in New York City depends on three nurses, two clinic aides, three interns unlucky enough to draw night duty—and me. I head up the emergency service at the Animal Medical Center, the biggest and some think best veterinary facility in the world. Often called the "Mayo Clinic for animals," for pet-owning New Yorkers it's the only place in town open on a twenty-four hour basis.

It was well after midnight when I finished treating my last patient, a small poodle who had been badly bitten by a Doberman guard dog and suffered several broken ribs. The poodle, now out of danger, was resting comfortably in the intensive care unit. Finally, the large second-floor waiting room of the AMC with its twelve rows of plain wooden seats, was empty. Miguel, the porter, made a last round of the room, cleaning up random puddles left by nervous patients, his mop and bucket sending the sharp, concentrated smell of ammonia into every corner of the reception area. Except for an occasional bark or bay emanating from the patient wards, the hospital was quiet. I could go home.

We had handled over eighty cases this rainy Tuesday evening, everything from a Chihuahua puppy almost electrocuted by a chewed light cord, to a guinea pig we saved after its owner inadvertently sat on it. Not to mention the dogs hit by cars, the cats who hurled themselves off penthouse terraces or out of high-rise windows and the victims of the usual run of oddball accidents and routine ailments suffered by animals living in an urban environment.

The overnight intern had checked in half an hour ago, and I had dismissed my staff. Now, so exhausted the tips of my fingers ached, I leaned against the clinic reception desk, too tired even to return to my tiny office at the other end of the floor and exchange the dirty, blood-stained lab coat I wore for my old army jacket. I half-listened to Carmen, the night receptionist, chattering on the phone in Spanish to her boyfriend. It was a nightly marathon conversation, punctuated with sighs and giggles, while she idly flipped through the pages of a magazine, usually *Playgirl* or *Viva*.

Suddenly, the comparative quiet of the room was broken by a commotion on the ramp leading to the reception area, and three black men burst through the double doors of the waiting room, grunting under the weight of the burden they carried wrapped in a bloody blanket.

"Somebody help us!" the first man shouted. "We got a shot dog here!" He held the door open with his shoulder, almost dropping the front end of their bloody load, while the other two struggled to bring in the rear.

"Here, bring him in here and get him up on the table." I pointed to a treatment booth directly behind the reception desk. The overwhelming fatigue had miraculously disappeared. "Carmen, get me Dr. Hunnicutt and a clinic aide—fast!"

She ended her phone call abruptly and summoned the overnight intern and the aide over the loudspeaker, her voice echoing through the empty waiting room. "DOCTOR HUNNICUTT TO BOOTH FOUR, EMERGENCY! DOCTOR HUNNICUTT EMERGENCY, PUL-EAZE! CLINIC AIDE TO BOOTH FOUR WITH STRETCHER! CLINIC AIDE BOOTH FOUR, EMERGENCY!"

The first two men hoisted the dog, still in the blanket, onto the table. The third, the front of his tan windbreaker covered with blood, his face contorted by tears, lifted one fold of the blanket off the semiconscious German shepherd. The dog lay on his side, his paws neatly crossed. A bullet wound in his thigh soaked blood through his thick, dark fur. More blood trickled from his nose and mouth, and since there was no apparent head trauma, I had to look elsewhere for the cause. I gently rolled him half over on his back and discovered another wound through the left side of his chest. I lifted his upper lip and pressed his gum with my finger. It was pale pink, and his breathing was slightly labored.

"They shot 'im, just like that—*Bang! Bang!* He was jes' protectin' me an' they shot 'im!" The man in the windbreaker sobbed, tears streaming down his face and fogging his rimless glasses so he had to remove them.

Chris Hunnicutt and Tyler Brown, the clinic aide, came down the staff corridor at a run with an IV rig and a steel rolling stretcher.

"Gunshot," I told Chris, and inserted a Jelco catheter into the cephalic vein in the dog's right leg. "He's badly hurt, but it may not be fatal if we work fast. Let's just try and get him stabilized."

Chris hooked the plastic bag of life-saving fluids to the IV rig, and I connected the long, transparent tube to the catheter so that the lactated Ringer's solution immediately began to flow into the shepherd's vein. I filled a syringe with steroids and injected it directly into the catheter followed by 5 cc's of Keflex, an antibiotic.

"When did this happen?" I asked the men while I worked.

The man in the windbreaker was unable to speak. His friend, a tall, light-skinned, middle-aged man answered for him. " 'Bout an hour ago. Cops come bangin' on Charlie's door lookin' for a coke dealer somebody said was in the building. They had the wrong apartment. You can plainly see it wasn't Charlie."

I glanced at Charlie. Slight, almost fragile, with close-cropped steel-gray hair, and mahogany skin stretched over high cheekbones—he looked to be about seventy with his eyeglasses on, maybe more. His friend was probably right. Dope hardly seemed his line.

"Charlie wasn't quick enough openin' the door," the man continued, "so they busted in. King here jumped on 'em, an' they shot 'im, not once, but twice. Then, when they see it's the wrong guy they got, they jes' leave 'im, poor dog, jes' leave 'im bleedin' all over the carpet. Charlie come get me, an' I help 'im get King down in the street. But there ain't no cabs uptown this time a night, so I go an' get Mr. Thompson here," he nodded at the snappily dressed younger man, who stood silently in the corner, "an' he bring us down in his car. Blood all over the backseat. Hope we ain't too late?"

The shepherd was in shock. The bullet in his thigh had caused a flesh wound, bloody, but not irreparable. It was the chest that concerned me. The crackling, gurgling sounds I'd heard through the stethoscope could indicate pulmonary hemorrhage, which would also account for the blood in the nose and mouth. We had to get him to intensive care as quickly as possible.

"Chris, Tyler, let's get him on the stretcher—fast!" Using the blanket as a hoist, we gently lifted the dog onto the rolling steel table and folded the blanket's bloody ends over him.

Before we could push it into the corridor, the old man leaned over the stretcher and stroked the big dog's head with his bony hand, burying his face in the shepherd's neck. "Why they do this to you, boy? Why they do this?" He looked up at me, tears streaming down his hollow cheeks. "Ya gotta save 'im, Doc. Please save 'im—he's all I got!"

"We're gonna do our best," I told him, trying not to sound abrupt. But every second counted. "I'll be back to talk to you as soon as I can."

With Tyler trotting alongside holding up the IV rig, Chris Hunnicutt and I ran the rolling table down the staff corridor, behind the clinic booths and through the long ward hall toward ICU.

"Shouldn't we X-ray and see where the bullet is?" Chris asked.

"Not the way he's breathing. He could go sour in minutes. We want to stabilize him, not stress him. If we X-ray, we have to turn him this way and that. He could fade while we're doing it. We might know where the bullet is—but diagnostics won't help a dead dog."

Chris was a first-year intern from Texas. A shaggy-haired fellow with an unkempt reddish-blond beard that made him look older and much wiser than his twenty-three years. But he was quick and bright. He listened carefully and absorbed what I said. Though as yet he'd had little experience with emergency medicine, a few more months at the AMC handling cases like this one and he'd be an expert.

We banged the stretcher through the swinging ICU door. "Got a gunshot here, let's get crackin'!" I announced as we rolled into the room. Penny Soames, the ICU nurse, was adjusting the catheter on my poodle with the broken ribs. She gave the little dog an extra affectionate pat and quickly closed the door on his upper-row cage.

"Penny, let's put a jug cath in this guy and clean and clip these wounds. He's lost a lot of blood. We may have to transfuse him. Chris, get a hematocrit and see where we are."

Penny swung into action. The best nurse in the hospital, she worked as surely and deftly as any doctor on the staff. She inserted a catheter into the jugular vein on the left side of the shepherd's neck, removed the old one from his leg and reattached the IV to the new catheter. Within seconds, she was clipping the fur and cleaning the chest wound with Betadine scrub. "I thought you'd gone home to get your beauty rest, Steve."

"Yeah, but I knew you couldn't live without me, so I came back." I winked at her.

Penny's whole existence was wrapped up in this small room, with its rows of cages filled with critically ill animals. An androgynous-looking girl with a thin, pretty face, she seemed to prefer the comparative loneliness of overnight duty in ICU to the hurlyburly of a day job. She was very young, no more than twenty-one or -two, and I once questioned her about the lack of social life working nights dictated. Lately, I was finding that curtailment more and more difficult, and I usually finished at midnight.

"I've got my animals," she had said, smiling shyly. "That's all I really want."

Chris drew blood from the dog's leg, put it in a narrow glass tube and spun it in the centrifuge. He would measure the hematocrit, the volume of red cells present in the sample. "It's low, Steve," he held up the tube to the light. "But not as bad as I thought. He's got a crit of 22."

I breathed a sigh of relief. Normal hematocrit for a dog is 40 to 45 percent. Though 22 meant the shepherd had hemorrhaged significantly, he didn't require a transfusion. We'd monitor him closely every two or three hours and if the crit fell below 15,

we'd give him blood. Without X rays, we were literally working
in the dark. We didn't know where the bullet in the chest had
lodged or the extent of the damage it had done. But our job was
to stabilize the dog sufficiently, so that surgical services could take
over in the morning, X-ray him and perform whatever surgery
was needed.

Penny was clipping and cleaning the wound on his flank, when
the dog moaned softly. "Good fella," she whispered to him. "I'm
cleaning this up so you'll feel better, you'll see. What's his name,
Steve?"

"King, I think. Didn't have much time to talk with the
owner."

"OK, King, almost finished." She threw the dirty blood-soaked
cotton swab in the trash basket and stroked the shepherd's head.
He was still shocky. The fluids and steroids would help that, but
his breathing was raspy, and that worried me.

"Let's get him into the oxygen. Chris, give me a hand here."

Penny opened the door to the oxygen unit in the corner of the
room and held the IV rig while Chris and I carefully lifted the
wounded shepherd and laid him in the larger of the two com-
partments. If oxygen didn't ease the breathing, we'd have to do a
chest tap. Five minutes would tell the story.

While we waited, Penny attended to a beagle recovering from
heart surgery. His mournful howl competed with Joe Cocker's
sweet, hoarse voice singing "You Are So Beautiful," coming from
the small radio perched on the EKG unit. Chris Hunnicutt sat on
the treatment table, swinging his legs and reading *People* magazine. If he was lucky, King would be the only major case of the
night and Chris would spend the next seven hours with Penny,
watching over the sick and wounded already in ICU and the
three wards down the hall. But that wasn't the way it usually
happened. As with humans, the wee hours of the morning always
brought a fight for life, or accidents, to many animals in the city,
and if their owners knew about us and cared enough, they were
brought here.

ICU is the backbone of the Animal Medical Center. In this
room, critical cases are monitored and treated twenty-four hours a

day, by three shifts of nurses. Unfortunately, the comparatively small room isn't big enough. The two rows of large and small cages against the three walls and in the tiny anteroom can hold only thirty patients, and my greatest frustration working nights is to run back to ICU with a bleeding or badly injured animal, only to find those cages filled. Then it becomes a question of triage— who's well enough to be sent to a regular ward? Sometimes, no one is, and I'm pushed to make a decision. Which animal no longer needs oxygen? Which one won't have a seizure? Which one can make it till morning without being constantly watched?

Many of the cages have been donated by grateful clients and have brass plaques on them with inscriptions like, "In Memory of Sam and Squeaky—John and Irene Loftus," or "In Memory of Ollie, God's Perfect Dog—P. J. Greene." But even if the room were twice as large, with twice the number of cages donated, it wouldn't be sufficient.

"OK, let's have a look at this guy. He's had enough oxygen to make the difference."

Chris jumped off the table and opened the door to the unit. "The bleeding from his nose's stopped," he said, kneeling by the still inert shepherd.

I put my stethoscope to the dog's chest and listened carefully. His breathing had eased considerably. That didn't mean there wasn't pulmonary hemorrhage, but we wouldn't have to tap his chest, at least not now. I looked around the room for a vacant lower cage, where we kept large animals. They were, of course, all filled. Can't move the Doberman who just had kidney surgery, or the mutt knifed in a mugging this afternoon. Ah, the collie mix. She slept peacefully with a cast on her hind leg. Brought in last night after a car hit her, she'd probably be released tomorrow.

"Chris, get Tyler and take Elsa to B-Ward."

He called for the clinic aide, and together they eased the big collie out of her cage, hoisted her onto the rolling stretcher and moved her down the hall to her new accommodations.

Penny laid a fresh paper lining on the bottom of the vacated cage. Though we would keep the shepherd in oxygen for the next several hours, the cage would be ready. Because of shock, the dog had to be kept warm, so we carefully arranged heat lamps in the oxygen unit to keep his body temperature constant and pulled the IV tube through a hole in the top of the unit and attached it to the stand.

"Keep a close eye on him," I instructed Chris. "If the breathing goes bad again after he's in the cage, throw him in the oxygen, and if that doesn't work, you'll have to do a tap."

"Oh, Christ," Chris muttered under his breath.

"You can do it," I reassured him. A chest tap involved inserting a needle on a syringe through the muscles of the chest wall between the ribs and withdrawing air, or blood if there was hemorrhaging, to relieve the pressure on the lungs. "Penny's here; she'll help you." Penny raised her eyes to heaven. Another intern she'd have to teach his trade.

Now that the shepherd was, for the moment, out of danger, the spurt of energy that had carried me through the last half hour left. I was bone tired. "OK, kids, I bid you a fond adieu. I'm gonna talk to the client and then home. It's way past my bedtime."

"Don't stay up all night watching the Late Show." Penny knew of my addiction to old movies. It was the only way I could turn my head off after eight hours of animal mayhem at the AMC.

"I'll try not to." In truth, I'd been looking forward to *Beau Geste*, with Gary Cooper. By now, it was probably half over.

The three men were sitting on the long bench next to the cashier, the old man in the middle, his head in his hands. They jumped up in unison as I came toward them.

"As of now, he's stable," I announced. "The chest wound is serious, and we still don't know how much damage the bullet did. But at least his breathing's eased and his vital signs are OK. I'm sure he'll make it till morning; then they can X-ray and do the necessary surgery. His chances for recovery are good, I think."

The old man took both of my hands in his and squeezed them tightly. "You saved my dog's life. I thanks you for that. More than I can say, I thanks you."

"How much we owe you?" The younger man, Mr. Thompson,

the driver, spoke for the first time. He was about thirty-five, expensively dressed in gray flannel trousers, a white silk shirt and a brown, glove-leather jacket. "Don't you worry none about the money. Whatever it costs, it costs!" From the inside pocket of his jacket, he pulled the biggest wad of hundred-dollar bills I'd ever seen and flipped through them for emphasis. Most of the bills looked so new, I wondered if they were real.

"I can only give you an estimate now of $350. The final bill will depend on the extent of surgery done and the length of the dog's stay. You can pay half of it now and the rest when you pick him up."

Thompson peeled four crisp bills from the roll. "We pay all of it now. If Charlie needs more, he just come to me."

"Fine," I said, the possible source of Mr. Thompson's income flashing through my mind. But that was his business; I was anxious to settle it and go home. I filled out a case record for King and led the three men to the cashier's booth. Jonelle, the night cashier, was sound asleep behind the steel bars of her enclosure. I rapped a bar with my pen and woke her up. "Jonelle, these gentlemen are going to pay you in cash. Give them the usual receipt, please."

"I thanks you again for savin' my King. The Lord will bless you for it!" Charlie grabbed my hand again.

"You're welcome, Mr. Taylor. I'm glad I was able to help, he's a good dog. Now, here's a phone number you can call tomorrow to see how he's doing, or if you want, you can call me tomorrow night. My name is Kritsick, Dr. Steve Kritsick." I wrote the numbers on a card for the old man.

I looked at the big clock over the reception desk. It was almost two. Waves of fatigue washed over me. I took off my stained lab coat, threw it down the laundry chute and retrieved my army fatigue jacket and gym bag from the office closet. If I hurried, I might still catch the end of *Beau Geste,* the part where Ray Milland and Robert Preston give Gary Cooper the Viking's funeral.

Chapter 2

The setting sun reflected off the windows of the Rockefeller Institute residence building like an orange neon ball, casting long shadows down York Avenue. A block south, I threaded my way through the stalled stream of five o'clock traffic, as the cars, like one great automated slug, futilely tried to turn onto East River Drive at 62nd Street. The suburban-bound commuters seemed more impatient and aggressive than usual, honking their horns with angry insistence, as if that in itself would propel them out of the jam and onto the drive. Oblivious to the frantic whistle blowing and flailing arm motions of the brown-uniformed traffic director stationed perilously in the middle of the street, the cars crept well beyond the corner, making it impossible to reach the curb without climbing over bumpers.

I chose a nonthreatening red Volkswagen with a faded peace symbol on its windshield, stepped up on the bumper and leapfrogged to the sidewalk. The bearded driver burst out of the car shaking his fist. "What the hell you think you're doin', man?" he screamed.

"Trying to get to work, mister. Just trying to get to work," I called over my shoulder, giving him a two-fingered peace sign. I sprinted down 62nd Street, past the Mobil gas station, then twenty yards farther, under the concrete canopy and through the automatic glass doors of the eight-story, semimodern building on the East River that houses the Animal Medical Center.

"Hey, Doctor Steve! How are ya?" Amelia, the lobby receptionist, called brightly from behind her high desk. "Crazy out there, right?"

"Awful!" I agreed.

She leaned over the desk and whispered confidentially, "Full moon, all the nuts is out. You watch, it's gonna be wild tonight. Lottsa crips. Always when it's full moon the crips come." Amelia was Cuban, and her English was pretty good, but every once in a while, a word like creep became "crip."

"It couldn't be any worse than last night. If it is, I'm gonna look for other work." I signed the night register, blew her a kiss and raced up the staff stairway to the second floor, hoping Amelia's prediction was wrong.

The corridor connecting the patient wards, surgery and the ICU with the clinic booths bustled with the shift change—nurses bound for home, interns and residents bound for night lectures, staff doctors headed as far away as possible from the constant cacophony of meows, barks, howls and baying.

I sped down the narrow hallway behind the nine clinic booths toward the two-by-four room I used as a combination office-locker. Suddenly, there he was. I ran right into him, or rather he ran into me, the peak of his deerstalker hat almost piercing my armpit. R. J. Osbourne was Director and Chief of Staff of the AMC. He was an intense man whose every waking moment was involved with the hospital. It was his wife, his lover, his life and seemingly his only reason for being. The position gave him an enormous amount of power in the profession and I guess defeated whatever loneliness he may have felt. Through a network of spies and favorites, R.J. was aware of any slight, slur, or incursion in his fiefdom. He made it his business to know his staff's every move, personally and professionally, as he scurried through the hospital's halls like Alice's White Rabbit, always in a hurry, always late—usually for a crucial meeting with yet another "friend of the hospital."

Because I worked nights, I was able to steer clear of much of the AMC's politics, which as in most large institutions, were rampant. Still, R.J., out of the corner of his eye and ear, managed to keep track of my activities. Mantled in his hail-fellow-just-one-of-the-boys disguise, he peered up at me from under his hat. "Steve, howsa boy? Heard you had a real tough one last night, but you pulled him through. Good work! Love to talk with you more, but I'm on my way to drinks with some ver-ry big money and I'm late. Just keep up the good attitude, boy. That's what really counts, good attitude!"

I hate being called "boy," I'm too old and too tall. But with R.J. Osbourne, I had no choice. He put his hand to his hat peak in a salute and was gone down the hall.

The cubicle I called an office contained a desk, a phone and a closet already filled with ancient files, a ladder and cartons of obsolete textbooks. Never mind, it had a lock on it. I had exchanged my fatigue jacket and gym bag for a fresh white lab coat, hung my stethoscope around my neck and locked the closet door, when the beeper attached to my belt went off with its high-pitched squawk: "DOCTOR KRITSICK ON 268. DR. KRITSICK, 268, PUL-EAZE!" It was phone time. Every doctor at the AMC has a half hour of phone time each day, when he or she can be reached by clients to answer questions about the condition of their pets. This was mine.

"Hello, Doctor Cryptic?"

"Kritsick."

"Yes, well this is Mrs. Farrentino, Angelo's mother? How is he?"

"Angelo?" I quickly rummaged through the yellow sheets describing each patient and how the animal had been treated by the day service after I had admitted it to the hospital. I spotted Farrentino, Angelo, a six-year-old Yorkshire terrier.

"Angelo's just fine, Mrs. Farrentino. Surgery removed forty-five cents from his stomach and he's doing real well now."

"Oh, my poor baby!"

"We knew from the X rays last night he'd swallowed the change. We just didn't know how much. The weight of it formed a little pocket in his stomach. There was no way he was going to pass it, so we had to operate."

"Oh, my poor baby!"

"No need to worry, Mrs. Farrentino, he's in ICU now and—"

"ICU—intensive care! Oh, my God!"

"We always try to put an animal in ICU after surgery so it can be monitored until it's stable."

"He's not stable?"

"Mrs. Farrentino, I assure you he is stable. In fact, he'll probably be able to go home tomorrow, and you'll be forty-five cents
richer."

"How can you make a joke? It's not funny, Doctor Cryptic!"

"Kritsick. I'm sorry, it was a bad joke, Mrs. Farrentino. I just
want you to know your dog is really OK. I'll go back to ICU myself and check him again. If you like, you can call me later tonight."

"That's very nice of you. Thank you, Doctor Cripick."

"Kritsick!"

Most of the calls were like that, routine. Just telling clients how
the animal was and when he/she/it could go home. King, the
shepherd gunshot case from last night had been operated on and
both bullets were successfully removed. The dog was resting
comfortably and would be released at the end of the week. When
I called his owner to give him the good news, Charlie Taylor
blessed me enough to last a lifetime.

But I didn't get the chance to enjoy his blessings. The clinic
area was absolutely jumping. Almost every one of the waiting
room's sixty wooden seats was occupied by all manner of man,
woman and beast. Barking Dobermans, howling beagles, yapping
Chihuahuas, mewing, meowing and screaming cats, squawking
parrots and any number of quieter, caged and unseen creatures,
waited their turn in one of the eight treatment booths.

I checked into the "night pharmacy," so called because, when
the regular pharmacy closes at 11:00 P.M., we have to rely on the
drugs and supplies in the glass cabinets lining the walls of this
small room. Actually, it isn't a room at all. It's a windowless,
doorless passageway between treatment booths 6 and 7. And it
serves as much more than a pharmacy; it's the gathering place
and communications center for all those on clinic duty, day or
night. When clients register at the desk, the patients' records are
pulled from the files by the receptionist, put on a clipboard and
placed on the counter, just inside the night pharmacy doorway.
As a doctor finishes seeing a patient, he or she brings the record
up to date, takes it to the cashier, then returns to the doorway,

picks up the next case and loudly heralds the client and patient from the waiting room into a treatment booth. Just to keep things straight—*clients* are the people, *patients* are the animals.

The counter was stacked with waiting clipboards. Should I choose an interesting one, or should I go in order and set a good example for the interns? Usually, I followed the order in which clients were received, but sometimes my eye lit on a particularly nifty case, and I'd grab it. Not tonight; we were too busy to do anything but take them as they came.

I'd resigned myself to a case of flea infestation, when I heard an unmistakable voice behind me, warm and husky like Margaret Sullavan's, the object of my across-the-grave affection ever since I'd seen her in *The Shop Around the Corner* on the Late Show. Only this wasn't Margaret Sullavan, it was Kate Gilchrist, a second-year intern, who not only sounded like Sullavan, but reminded me of her in other ways. Maybe it was the clear intensity of her enormous blue eyes, or the straight, sun-streaked blond hair, cut just above the shoulders, and the bangs that tumbled across her forehead. It was hard to tell. Perhaps, it came down to her seeming unavailability. At work we were colleagues—friends. We laughed and joked, and she was always warm, if not outright affectionate. But oddly enough, the camaraderie we shared the few nights each month she was on my service never went any further. Not that I didn't try. Like every other single guy on staff, as well as some of the married ones, I'd asked her to have a drink or dinner when we weren't working, but with no success. Finally, fearing I'd wreck our working relationship by becoming a pest, I stopped asking. That seemed to suit Kate just fine.

"And how are you this gorgeous moonlit night?" She reached across me and picked up her clipboard from the counter, sending the light, fresh smell of the perfume she always wore up my nostrils and straight to my heart.

"Never better, now that you're here. I thought Chris Hunnicutt was on again, doing a double. How come you're working?"

"Chris thinks he has the flu, so you lucked out and got me."

I crossed myself, and she laughed. "Why do you do that? Chris is pretty good."

"They're all pretty good, but you're better." I truly meant that. Kate was a superb veterinarian, one of the best interns I'd ever worked with. She was a natural. Her medical competence was finely complemented by a caring warmth that was immediately transmitted to the animals she treated as well as to their owners. Soon she would begin her residency in cardiology under John Garth, who was not only the head of the AMC cardiology department, but one of the country's leading veterinary cardiologists. Kate was planning to specialize in feline heart problems and would do well. In the end, probably a lot better than Margaret Sullavan.

She fingered the stethoscope around her neck as she studied the case record on the clipboard. "Jesus, Steve, this one looks like a dilly. I may need your help. It's a kitten with a needle stuck in its palate."

"Call me if you want me. I'll be in four with the flea circus."

I stepped toward the waiting room and loudly called, "Mulkowski! Peter Mulkowski!" There was no response. I called again, trying to make myself heard over the howling beagle. "Mulkowski! Peter Mulkowski!" Finally, a large woman wearing a navy polyester pants suit shuffled toward me. The big metal rollers in her hair were barely masked by a kerchief she had tied around her head, turban style. At the end of the leash, in front of her, was a sad-eyed shepherd-collie mix, who walked four steps, sat down and scratched, then walked four steps again. I could see the fleas jumping off his back and immediately began to itch.

"Peter Mulkowski?"

"Nah, Peter's drivin' the cab. I drive it during the day. I'm Mrs. Mulkowski. This is Jack. He rides with us in the cab—protection, ya know. But now he's got these fleas so bad he's makin' us crazy, and I think I'm gettin' 'em too." She scratched her side to demonstrate.

"Come in here, let's have a look." I motioned them into Booth 4 and lifted Jack up onto the table. He was a sweet, patient dog, who had the face and head of a shepherd, but unfortunately, the long thick coat of a collie. I parted the hairs around his neck and then his back and under his tail. There were fleas everywhere.

They danced off his fur onto the table and up my arm. God, how I hate them!

"Have you given him a flea bath?"

"What d'ya think I am, a dummy? Of course I gave 'im a flea bath. He's had two baths. They don't work. He's OK for a day or so, then they come right back."

"I hate to have to tell you this, Mrs. Mulkowski, but they're probably in your house. You're gonna have to use an insecticide bomb to get rid of them. They're probably in your taxi too, so you'll have to bomb that."

"How can we? We use it all the time."

"I don't know, Mrs. Mulkowski, you'll have to figure out a time. Fleas lay eggs, and you've got to get the eggs. Now, I'll give you a medicated shampoo for Jack and a flea collar. Give him a bath, then when everyone, including Jack, is out of the house, use the bomb. Keep the flea collar on him. It doesn't prevent fleas, but it helps. And don't forget the taxi."

"That's all I need—fleas!" Mrs. Mulkowski moaned. "It's not enough we work twenty-four hours a day, but we have to have fleas. Maybe I should go on welfare, like some of those cheats out there. You know some of those bums never work a day in their lives, never a day."

I didn't know which cheats she was referring to, but I wanted to get her, Jack and the fleas out of the booth as quickly as possible. "Welfare won't stop fleas, Mrs. Mulkowski. Jack has to have a shot of cortisone because he's had an allergic reaction to them. It'll help the itching. Would you hold him for a minute, while I prepare the injection?"

Mrs. Mulkowski held the dog at arm's length. While I was administering the needle, I noticed a flea jump from the dog's neck to the front of her open-collared jacket and down her ample bosom. I said nothing.

"OK, that should take care of it. Why don't you and Jack wait outside in the corridor and I'll get the medicated shampoo and the collar for you."

I put the dog on the floor and handed his lead to his mistress. The minute they were in the hall, I closed the door to the booth and sprayed the table, the floor and myself with insecticide. I itched all over. Goddamned fleas! With my luck, I'd leave the hospital tonight and get right into Peter Mulkowski's taxi.

The sliding door on the other side of the booth, which led to the staff corridor, opened and Kate Gilchrist stuck her head in. "Steve, I think I do need you. The needle's really imbedded in the roof of the kitten's mouth. Been there since last Thursday!"

"Oh, Christ! All right, meet you in the prep room as soon as I pick up some stuff from the pharmacy."

"The bill will be thirty-five dollars. Thirty for the visit and five for the medication," I told Mrs. Mulkowski and handed her the shampoo and collar in a brown paper bag.

"Thirty-five dollars!" she howled. Her kerchief had come undone and was hanging off the metal rollers. "You've got to be kidding! Thirty-five dollars for fleas? What do you charge the welfare cheats? Nothing, I bet!"

"The same as you, Mrs. Mulkowski. Unless you're blind, or over sixty-five and indigent, this isn't a free clinic. It's a hospital, just like Lenox Hill or Mount Sinai, and it costs a great deal to run. Now, make sure you bathe him as soon as possible and don't forget the insect bomb and flea collar." There wasn't time to jabber with her about the inequities of New York's social structure. I left her holding the shampoo and scratching herself and ran down the staff corridor.

I found Kate Gilchrist in the surgery prep room. She had already begun to work on the kitten. Jonas Sidley, the surgical nurse, held the squirming, undernourished hank of gray and white fur on the exam table, while Kate pried open its mouth. The kitten, not more than ten weeks old, screamed loudly.

"Sorry it took me so long; politics got confused with fleas." I was still scratching.

"Would you believe she swallowed the needle five days ago? Been gagging, choking and screaming ever since, and they waited till now to bring her in." Kate leaned down and scanned the kitten's upper palate with a tiny flashlight. "Damn it! She's squirming so much, I can't see. Jonas, hold her tighter."

"I'm trying, Doctor Gilchrist. The little ones are harder than the big ones." Jonas bent over the table, steadying his hands by leaning on his elbows.

"I think we should tranq her." I drew up 1/10 of a cc of ketamine and injected it into the kitten's leg. She screamed even louder.

"There it is. I see it. Look, Steve." Kate tapped the back of the palate with a hemostat, indicating the needle. "Her mouth is so small and it's so far back, it'll be hard to get."

Even with the ketamine, the kitten continued to squirm and scream. The pain must've been intense. "Let's put her out," I said. "Jonas, get the anesthesia ready. I'll hold her."

Jonas pulled the halothane and oxygen tanks close to the table and hooked them up to an enormous nose cone. He put it over the kitten's face, but it was so big her entire body disappeared in it.

"Haven't we got a smaller cone?" I asked. "That one'd be right for a tiger."

Jonas produced a small nose cone, and the struggling kitten inhaled the gas. Finally, she was quiet. As I held her mouth open, Kate probed for the needle with the hemostat, beads of perspiration forming on her nose and upper lip.

"God, it's in deep. I'm touching it, but I can't grab it."

"Here, let me try. You hold her." I changed places with Kate. The kitten began to move and squeal. "Give her more gas, Jonas," I ordered.

He squeezed the black rubber bag above the tanks, and the kitten was still again. I probed the tender roof of her mouth until the pincer tips of the hemostat hit the needle. Kate was right; it was in very deep. I pressed down hard on one end so that the other end of the needle poked through the membrane. I grabbed it, but when I pulled it out, my heart sank. A long thread attached to the needle led down the back of the kitten's throat to the esophagus. I yanked on the thread gently, and the feeling at the other end was as if I'd hooked a big fish. "Damn! Kate, look at this."

The minute she saw the thread, she recognized the problem. "Do you think it's wound round her intestines?"

"Afraid so. It's been there too long not to be." The intestines work like an accordion, and with the movement, the thread could eventually cut through the intestinal wall. "I guess it's bad news for our little friend here. She's gonna need surgery."

"I have a feeling our little friend has had nothing but bad news since the day she was born. You should see what brought her in here." Kate shook her head in disgust. "Two teenage girls, both high as kites. The kitten belongs to the mother of one of them. When I told the kid where I thought the needle was, she said, 'That cat'll be all right. I already dropped it down the incinerator and it lived. It's got eight more lives to go.' To tell you the truth, Steve, if the poor thing does make it, I'd hate to give her back to those girls; she'll only be mistreated again. Look at her." Kate picked up the emaciated kitten and held it in the crook of her elbow. "She hasn't been fed, she's skin and bones. It's a wonder she's survived this long. The best thing we could do for her, probably, is put her to sleep. At least we'd know she wasn't suffering anymore." Her blue eyes clouded with anger. "Sometimes I wonder if I've chosen the right profession. You'd think after a year here I'd've toughened up. But it still makes me furious when we work so hard to save an animal and then we have to send it out there again to get beat up on. I don't think I'll ever get used to that, and if I can help it, I won't do it!"

"Don't you think I feel the same way? How many times have I said to myself, 'What's a nice Jewish boy doing in a place like this?' I could've been a gynecologist in a cushy practice, making my mother happy, and with a pile of dough to boot."

The anger slowly disappeared from her face, she smiled her Margaret Sullavan smile, and a funny little line appeared above her upper lip. I had seen it before and visualized it whenever I thought about Kate. It's odd, how you can find such a tiny physical attribute so attractive—the way someone holds her head, or raises an eyebrow, or in this case, that funny little line.

"Did you really want to be a gynecologist?" She seemed incredulous. "Steve Stunning a gynecologist? My, my, they would've been lined up around the block," she laughed.

"Nah, I always wanted to be a vet. Ever since I was fourteen and cleaned cages for Doctor Waters in Concord, Mass. In fact, I don't think being anything else ever entered my mind. I've always loved animals. Though gynecology undoubtedly has its compensations." I winked at her. "Ah, listen Kate, it's this place. It's like a pressure cooker. It burns you out. Don't you think it makes me a little crazy to have to deal with this kind of thing, night after night? At least you usually work days. It's different during the day. You've got all kinds of backup. You've got staff, you've got specialists. You see maybe ten, or at most fifteen, cases. At night, it's me and three interns. Sometimes there's one as good as you are. But mostly they're inexperienced or slow. They don't use their heads, and on a night like this, when I bet you we end up seeing seventy-five or eighty cases, I just want to kick 'em in the ass. Anyway, in a few years you'll be board certified in cardiology. Then you can go off to a nice, soft private practice where all the clients dress well and speak perfect English."

"Why don't you do that?" She asked with real interest.

"I did, and at the end of a year my eyes crossed, I was so bored."

"Well, so would mine." She crossed them to demonstrate.

"OK, enough said," I laughed. "Let's get that kitten into radiology and find out how bad it is."

Radiology was almost adjacent to the surgery prep room. We pushed open the heavy steel door and found Ito, the Japanese technician, scanning X rays on the light panel. I laid the drugged kitten on the X-ray table and donned a lead apron and gloves.

"Ito, this baby swallowed a needle. We need some quick pictures. No charge."

"How come no charge?"

"Because the people won't pay, and we need to know how much damage the thread has done!"

He asked no further questions. While Kate waited outside, I held the kitten on the table and Ito went into the lead-lined closet and activated the X-ray machine. Within three minutes, Kate was back in the room and we were looking at a film of the kitten's abdomen. The thread was indeed tightly interwoven in a criss-cross pattern.

"The only option is to cut that out." I looked at Kate.

"I know. There's no way those girls are going to come up with $300 for surgery on this kitten. I wouldn't even suggest it. I'm going to recommend putting her to sleep. I don't think they'll care. It'll probably be a relief." She lifted the unconscious kitten from the table and cradled it in her arms. "At least I'll be able to give you a little peace—finally," she whispered to it. "I'll put her in ICU for now and go and talk with them."

"Don't forget to have them sign the release," I reminded her.

"I won't. And, Steve—thanks for the help."

"Anytime. Aren't you glad I'm not a gynecologist?"

"I'll have to think about that." She smiled, and there was just the faintest trace of that funny little line.

Chapter 3

The windows of the narrow corridor behind the treatment booths looked out on the East River. It was dark now, and the lights on the 59th Street Bridge winked red, white and yellow, as a steady stream of traffic edged its way across to Queens. Sometimes, even after five years in New York, it was still hard for me to believe I was really here and this wasn't the dream residue of some movie I had seen as a kid at the Lexington Bijou.

Emily Addison told me I could be anything and do anything I wanted, if I just set my head to it. Emily was about forty then, I was fifteen. We sat in the cockpit of her Piper Cherokee, as she expertly banked and rolled the small plane through the clouds over Concord and Bedford, a million miles from Dr. Waters's veterinary clinic below. We were both employed by Dr. Waters, she as his "associate," I as his kennel boy. Her dogs, Harmon and Edgar, sat in the backseat of the plane, attentively watching over her shoulder every move she made. They were mutts. Edgar was a sheepdog-collie mix and Harmon, part German shepherd, part Irish setter. She had adopted them two years before, after they had been abandoned, and now they went everywhere with her. I liked to think that aside from me, they were her closest companions. Since I had never known anyone like Emily Addison, that she chose to pay attention to me and care at all about what I grew up to be, was then the joy and miracle of my life.

"If I'm gonna be a vet, I want to be as good as you are. I want to be the best," I told her earnestly.

"I don't know that I'm the best, but I'm not bad," she admitted. She took off her dark aviator glasses and turned to me and smiled so that her white teeth showed and her pale blue eyes crinkled at the corners. I hoped she didn't see that my cheeks had flushed when she looked at me. Emily was not beautiful, but she had a unique style that was perhaps, fifteen years ahead of its time. Her long, curly auburn hair was piled carelessly on top of her head and secured in a knot with a zig-zag series of tortoise-shell barrettes. She was of medium height and slender to the point of being slight, her body giving no outward indication of the tensile strength that allowed her to lift a hundred-pound dog onto the examining table with ease. She didn't seem to care much about her clothes, though they had a certain flair. She wore only what was practical and comfortable. Now that I think about it, Ralph Lauren has made a fortune copying the very things Emily ordered then, from the L. L. Bean catalog.

The one time I brought Emily home to dinner, my mother was possibly put off by her baggy corduroy trousers, linen shirt and safari jacket. But she finally agreed later, under pressure from me, that Dr. Addison was a "most unusual woman—striking, in her way." To me, she was that and much more. I looked at her tanned face that summer day two thousand feet in the air and thought she was nothing short of splendid. My heart pounded furiously, and the palms of my hands were suddenly damp and clammy. If only the plane never had to land, or better still, if only we could fly somewhere a thousand miles away, where no one knew us. We'd set up a clinic and she'd teach me everything she knew, and we'd live happily ever after—just Emily and me and untold numbers of sick and injured animals.

She interrupted my reverie. "Aside from all the technical stuff, being a good vet is caring. That's what it's all about, Steve. You have to care about every animal you treat as if it were your own. You have to love them. They know if you do and they respond, sometimes better than humans, I think. But you know, not all vets care. Some of them are in it just for the money." She banked the plane steeply, and we were out of the clouds. Now I could see the neat green, brown and yellow squares of planted Concord farms. They looked like an aerial map from my geography book.

Though she didn't say it, I knew she was talking about Dr. Waters. He was a 9-to-5 vet, who never would have qualified in the St. Francis of Assisi stakes. Even from my lowly kennel-boy vantage point, I could see that Waters's primary concern was the fees his clients paid. He never saw emergencies after office hours, even if a dog had been hit by a car right in front of his clinic, whereas Dr. Addison would make house calls and get up in the middle of the night, if necessary, to treat a sick cat.

Dr. Waters had been in practice for about twenty years. Most of that time he was the only vet in town, until Dr. Addison joined his clinic, and anyone who didn't like his methods had to drive thirty miles to see another vet. Waters was a businessman and he cut corners any way he could to save a buck. That's why he hired me. At twenty-five cents an hour, he couldn't go wrong. I was cheap labor. Real cheap. Every day after school and for three hours on Saturday and Sunday, I cleaned the cages and fed the animals. He gave me the job as a favor to my father, who hoped that working for Waters would increase the interest I'd already expressed in veterinary medicine and put my almost obsessive love for animals to good use.

Actually, if it hadn't been for Emily Addison, nothing would have turned me off quicker. Waters was a colorless man who probably had been born old and crotchety. His lack of personal warmth and charm was compounded by a physical trait that made him all the more unattractive. He cracked his knuckles as a kind of punctuation when he explained a diagnosis to a client, or gave an order to any member of his staff. He said it helped him to think, but Emily said she thought it was a form of masturbation.

Dr. Waters couldn't have cared less about my aspirations. I was there to clean cages, not to be inspired watching him in surgery. It was Emily who answered my incessant questions and it was Emily who made me think being a vet was the noblest, warmest, most wonderful profession in the world. In effect, Emily Addison was the first adult outside of my family who really noticed me and treated me as more than a set of legs and arms, good only to fetch and carry. In return, I idolized her.

But, I knew she wouldn't stay long. She was too good a vet for

Waters. Trained at Angell Memorial Animal Hospital in Boston, she was used to the best equipment and the best veterinary medicine practiced in the country. It was hard to understand why she chose to work in a dump like Dr. Waters's clinic. The waiting room looked like something Norman Rockwell might have chosen for an old *Saturday Evening Post* cover. Its dark wood-paneled walls were hung with prints of collies, shepherds and setters, by Gladys Emerson Cook. Reproductions of early-American wooden armchairs were scattered about the room. A tall wooden hat rack stood in the corner and a frayed and urine-stained hooked rug covered the wide-planked floor. However, the folksy atmosphere of the entrance was belied by the dingy unlit room downstairs where the animal cages were kept. Charles Dickens couldn't have conceived of anyplace more depressing. But the clients never saw that nor did they see the small, badly equipped surgery. Dr. Addison was always fighting with Waters about equipment, particularly about the glass hypodermic syringes he insisted on using again and again.

"For God's sake, this is 1965," she'd shout. "No one's used glass hypodermics since World War II. They're unsanitary and the needles are too big—they hurt!"

Once, when I was lurking about the treatment room, pretending to empty the trash basket so I could be near her, Emily picked up a glass hypodermic to give a dog a distemper shot and realized the needle was bent. She hurled it against the wall, where it shattered in a hundred pieces. Luckily, only the dog and I were in the room with her. If Waters had been there, amidst a great cracking of knuckles, he might have fired her, or worse, she might have just walked out. I knew something like that would happen soon and I dreaded it so much, I made compacts with God as I rode my bicycle to the clinic every day. "Please dear God, let Dr. Addison still be there. If you do, I promise I'll do anything. I won't play my records too loud. I won't be mean to Charlotte. I'll clean up my room. I'll be your best friend—just let her still be there!"

My deep affection and admiration for Emily had begun the year before, when I was fourteen and had only been working for Dr. Waters for two weeks. It was early on a Sunday morning, I had a key to the clinic and had gone immediately to the downstairs ward to clean the cages and feed their occupants, when I discovered Honey, the poodle in the last cage, had begun to whelp. She had already dropped the first puppy. I had never seen a birth before and I sat on the floor at the side of the cage and watched, mesmerized, as she chewed at the umbilical cord attaching her to her firstborn. When she had severed the cord, she began to lick the tiny mass of wet, black fur, no bigger than a mouse, as it lay perfectly still on the pile of shredded newspaper. But it was minutes before I realized the puppy hadn't moved. I was alone in the clinic. Panic grabbed my stomach when the new mother looked up at me and whimpered with what I was certain was a cry for help. I reached into the cage and gently lifted the puppy out and held it in the palm of my hand. It was cool to the touch, its little legs still in the fetal position, its eyes sealed shut. I would give artificial respiration, just as I had seen it done on television with humans. I turned the puppy, still in my palm, on its back, and under Honey's concerned gaze, opened its mouth and breathed into its lungs, once, twice, three times and then again, with no success. It never moved. When Emily arrived, she found me sitting cross-legged on the floor, holding the dead puppy against my chest, tears streaming down my face. She knelt beside me and took the heaviest burden I had ever carried from my hand.

"If only I'd known more, I could've saved it," I sobbed. "I breathed into it. I really tried, but it just wouldn't live."

Emily looked at the tiny, lifeless form briefly and laid it on the treatment table, wrapping it in a small white hand towel. "It was stillborn, Steve. There was nothing you could've done. Nothing either of us could've done." She put her arms around me and dried my tears with a red bandana she pulled from around her neck. "You've lost your first patient, Dr. Kritsick, that always hurts the most. No matter how many you lose after this, and unfortunately, you'll lose a lot, this is the one you'll always remember. But you tried. You did your very best with what was at hand and that's what counts. Now, blow your nose and let's see if Honey has some more in her."

She handed me the bandana and turned to see Honey drop another puppy. This one was squirming. She took a pair of surgical scissors from her jacket pocket and gave them to me. "You do the honors. Honey's gonna need a hand, she's got at least two others to come." She was palpating the poodle's belly as she talked. I clipped the cord, not too close to the navel, just as Emily instructed. Honey did the rest, eating the afterbirth, licking the puppy to wash it and then pushing it to her milk-heavy breast to suckle. Under Emily's watchful eye, I repeated the process three more times. Honey and I delivered a healthy litter of four squealing, hungry puppies. Dr. Addison gave the poodle an antibiotic shot to prevent a uterine infection, and I filled her bowl with a well-deserved dinner. From the look and sound of her brood, Honey would need all of her strength.

I was full of myself. In the short space of one Sunday morning, I had seen death and helped to bring life, all for the first time. It was kind of an epiphany. From that moment on, the course of my life was charted, irrevocably. Now even the loss of the first puppy didn't seem quite as tragic. I found a cigar box used for paper clips, emptied it, neatly placed my first patient inside and closed the lid. We buried the box in a shallow grave outside the clinic, marking it with a circle of small stones. I had never shared anything as important with anyone. As far as I was concerned, Dr. Emily Addison and I were now forever joined.

Sometimes after the clinic closed for the day, Dr. Addison would ask me to stop by her house for a Coke or a cup of tea. I never drank tea except when I was sick, and my mother always used tea bags. But Emily Addison brewed it from scratch, using Earl Grey tea. She was very specific about that; it had to be Earl Grey. I've drunk it since and it just tastes like strong tea, but then, it was the nectar of the gods. She lived alone with her two dogs in a small rented house in Lincoln. The furniture came with the house, but she had things scattered about that made it her own—an Indian blanket thrown over the arm of the chair in front of the fireplace, a small dhurrie rug covering the worn carpet under the coffee table near the couch, stacks of books and records on every table surface and framed photographs on the mantel.

One photo in a silver frame particularly interested me. It was a picture of Emily and a young man, taken when she was in her twenties. They were standing in front of a small plane. They wore jeans and matching plaid shirts. Her hair was long, to her shoulders. The young man had his arm around her, and they both were smiling and squinting at the sun. Once, she saw me studying it and said softly, "That was my husband."

I felt as if I'd been caught rummaging through her drawers. "I didn't know you were married," I stammered.

"It was a very long time ago. He was killed in an accident." She quietly closed the drawer, and I asked nothing further. Finding out more about Emily became a game to me. The rules were, I asked no questions. I could only piece together information from whatever crumbs she chose to drop along the way of our relationship, though I was dying to know all about her. She seemed to have few friends, and our conversations centered around the events at Dr. Waters's clinic, books, her days as an intern at Angell—and me. She loved classical music and opera and always had a record going while we talked. It was my introduction to Mozart, Bach, Brahms and Wagner. At home, my parents never played anything but elevator music, and I had previously confined myself to Bob Dylan and the Beatles, behind the closed door of my room.

Those were her three passions, I guess, animals, music and flying. She shared them with me generously, and with the usual selfishness of a fourteen-year-old boy, I was grateful then that there was no one else to take up her time or distract her from me. Though, at times, I had vivid fantasies about her personal life, even endowing her with a secret love affair, star-crossed, of course.

I needed her encouragement. I needed her to open the door, just a crack, to the possibilities of the world that lay beyond. My perceptions of Emily were all tangled with my own adolescent insecurities and desires. What I thought of, then, as her stalwart independence and slightly peculiar self-sufficiency, in reality, may have been a deep loneliness that I was able to relieve a little with my eager but unthreatening attention. I suppose that was a fair

enough deal. In the years since, I've met many people in the profession who communicate better with animals than they do with
humans. That's why they chose to become vets. It's not the right
reason, and I don't believe Emily began that way, but by the time
I met her, I think she had become one of those people.

When I could, I led her into conversations about Angell. I had
already made up my mind that that was where I would intern
after I finished vet school and I wanted to know everything about
it. If only it were possible to jump inside her head like a little
sponge and soak up all the visual images of the place that she had
stored there. When she spoke of it, she made the hospital sound
like an animal version of Massachusetts General. It had hustle
and bustle and glamour. There were night emergencies and rare
diseases and exotic animals and overnight "shifts" and operating
"greens," buzz words with which I've since become too familiar.
But then, they conjured up a picture of excitement and life-
threatening drama that had absolutely no relationship to Dr. Waters's veterinary clinic. More than anything, I needed to see it
with my own eyes.

After six months of cleaning cages every day, I had managed to
squirrel away twenty dollars. It was earmarked for a birthday
present for my sister, Charlotte, but my new plan was suddenly
much more important. I would take Dr. Addison to lunch in
Boston, and in return, she would show me Angell from the inside.
I had never taken anyone to lunch in Boston, much less spent
twenty dollars, so I expected she would be as excited as I was
when I offered the invitation. Instead, her face fell. "I'd have to
dress up." She ran her hands down her navy corduroy L. L. Bean
trousers. "I can't wear these to lunch in Boston."

"You don't have to dress up much," I assured her. "It's just
lunch and we don't have to go anyplace really fancy." I had been
thinking about the Parker House, which my mother said was the
best restaurant in Boston. She must have seen the disappoint-
ment in my eyes. She tapped her foot for a minute. "Can't have
you moping around here looking like a sick hound. I'll throw
something together that's presentable."

I was overjoyed. Now it was only a matter of living until Satur-

day. We agreed that I would pedal my bicycle to her house and
then we'd drive her pickup into Boston. When the day finally
came, I spent an hour primping in front of the mirror. I changed
my tie four times, ending up with a navy and red regimental
stripe belonging to my father. I didn't have a whole suit, so I wore
gray flannel trousers and the navy-blue blazer my mother had
given me for my birthday, not quite a year before. I had grown
two inches since then, so my wrists hung out from the sleeves. I
tried, unsuccessfully, to shoot the cuffs of my shirt so the knobby
bones wouldn't show, and I carefully tucked the twenty dollars in
my new wallet, another present from last year I hadn't used.

When I pedaled up to her house, Dr. Addison was standing on
the steps waiting for me. In her own special way, she too had
dressed for the occasion. She wore beige gabardine slacks and a
beige turtleneck sweater under a belted brown suede jacket.
Around her neck, she had flung a white silk aviator's scarf. Her
curly auburn hair, instead of being randomly piled on her head,
was now neatly caught in a twist at the nape of her neck. And for
the first time since I'd known her, she wore lipstick. All in all,
Emily Addison looked if not glamorous, then certainly dashing.
She caught my goggle-eyed expression.

"Well, a date's a date." She smiled slyly. "I decided to dress
for it."

The day was glorious, warm for mid-October. The events of it
became a slide show that I would replay in my head for the next
year. The sun dappled the leaves, already turned red and orange
from the first frost, as we drove down Route 2 to Boston in
Emily's blue pickup. My father had made a reservation for us at
the Parker House, so when we arrived, the head waiter escorted
us to our table with great flourish.

We ordered clam chowder and then sautéed bay scallops, the
sweetest and tiniest I had ever eaten. Emily seemed to be having
a wonderful time, and I felt very grown up, surprisingly at ease in
my new role as host. Of course, she always made me feel that
way. Emily treated me as an equal, not as a kid. To her, we were
good friends laughing and chatting about shared experiences.
When we overheard the man at the next table loudly and preten-

tiously ordering wine, we looked over just in time to see him crack his knuckles exactly the way Dr. Waters did. We laughed so hard, I began to choke. Emily made me raise my arms above my head and whacked me on the back.

"Here, take some water." She handed me the glass and wiped the tears from her face. "We just can't get away from him, can we?" When she said that we both dissolved again into spasms of uncontrollable giggles.

"It's all right for you," she gasped, "but it's rather unseemly for old Dr. Addison to be giggling at the Parker House."

"You're not old anything. You're wonderful, Emily." Impulsively, I leaned over and kissed her on the cheek. She took my hand in hers and held it tightly.

"You're a bright, warm and sensitive boy, Steve, and I've come to care about you very much. In fact, if it hadn't been for you, I think I would have left Waters months ago. I've never said this to you before because I think the experience you're getting will be valuable to you later on and I don't want to discourage you, but now I have to say it; Waters is not only a mean-spirited man, he's a rotten vet."

"I know that, Emily, do you think I'm stupid? I have eyes and I can see how you work and how he works. What I've never understood is why you came to his clinic in the first place. You're too good for him." I had broken my rule and asked a flat-out question, but now I didn't think Emily would mind.

"Oh, it's a long story, Steve. Life has a way of making odd twists and turns, and unless you're a very strong swimmer, you get carried along until you suddenly wake up one day working for a Dr. Waters. That wasn't the way I'd planned it—not at all. You know I was married. Well, I met my husband when I was interning at Angell. He had just finished his residency in pediatrics at Mass. General, and we were married when I completed my internship. Thom, that was his name, was offered a position with a large medical group in Denver, and I found a place there in a good veterinary practice. He was a flyer. I think he loved planes almost more than he loved medicine, and when he taught me to fly, it became something we could share completely. He had an old Piper Cub, and after a year, we gave ourselves a great present and traded it in for a Beechcraft. Oh, it was a lovely plane. Our dream was to move to Alaska. I thought I could start a good practice there, and Thom could be a flying doctor. Neither of us liked big cities and we thought we'd really be needed in Alaska. It was a romantic dream, but we were young and we loved each other very much, so anything was possible. After five years, we had saved almost enough money to make the move. Life was just exquisite. I couldn't have asked for more on my plate, and then whammo, it happened." I noticed the pain reflected in Emily's eyes and remembered the accident she had mentioned when I was looking at the picture on the mantel.

"Maybe you don't want to talk about it, Emily. You don't have to."

"I think it might be good if I do. I haven't talked about it to anyone in years. Usually, I try not to think about it. But somehow, Steve, I'd like you to know." She picked up a fork and drew lines with it on the tablecloth. "Anyway, Thom had promised to fly a friend of ours up to Aspen to look at some property. He called me at the office to ask if I'd like to sneak away and come with them. But I had a heavy case load that day and I couldn't." She made deeper lines with the fork. "That was the last time I spoke with him. It was early spring, and storms came up in the mountains, out of nowhere." She paused and seemed to look straight through me. "They didn't find the plane for three days."

"God, Emily, I'm sorry."

"It was a long time ago. When it happened, I thought my life was finished and, in one way, it was. But you go on. When I talk about it now, it's as if I'm speaking of someone else. You know how it is when you hold the negatives of old snapshots up to the light—you recognize the general shape of people, but you can't see any distinct features. That's how those years seem to me now. The pain is still there, but it's no longer sharp."

"Did you stay in Denver?"

"For a while. I had my work, thank God. But I found I was making a blanket of memories of the places we'd been and the things we'd done. I wrapped myself so tightly in it, I was smothering. Truly, some mornings I'd wake up feeling the air was being sucked out of my lungs and I couldn't breathe. So after three years of being miserable and feeling sorry for myself, I decided to get as far away from Denver as possible. I heard of an opening in Washington, D.C., and grabbed it. It was a nice practice run by a father and son. I stayed for five years and then got itchy again. As I told you, I don't like big cities. I saw an ad for the position with Dr. Waters in the *Veterinary Journal* and decided coming back to New England might be the right thing to do. I hadn't counted on Waters's antediluvian methods, or his charming personality." She smiled wryly. "So my young friend, there you have it, as briefly as possible, the story of Emily Addison. Hardly the stuff of movies."

She put the fork down and stared at the tablecloth without saying anything. She needed the moment to give what she had been talking about time to settle back into that mental compartment in which she'd kept it neatly tucked for so long.

I was slightly uncomfortable. Pleased on the one hand to have some of my questions about Emily answered at last, but on the other hand, I felt incapable of offering her any real comfort. Not that she wanted or expected any from me. I just wished I could've said something, or done something that would have wiped it all away for her. I think, for the first time, I was aware of the awful separateness of people, even if they're very close.

"Well," she said finally, pulling us both back, "did you forget? We're here for a purpose. We've got very important fish to fry this afternoon, and if we don't get started soon, it'll be too late in the day."

Almost on cue, the waiter arrived and presented me with the check on a silver tray. Emily grabbed for it. "Let me take you, Steve, else you'll be cleaning cages for Waters another whole year to pay for it."

"No," I insisted. I already had my twenty dollars out and laid it proudly on the check. There was barely enough left over for the ten percent tip my father had told me to leave. I couldn't let Emily Addison pay. Not only did I badly want to impress her with my grown-up savoir faire, but after all, this was in a way a business lunch, and now the business was at hand.

As if she were taking a Moslem to Mecca, Emily drove me in the pickup along Longwood Avenue, Boston's medical ghetto, pointing out the Harvard Medical School, Children's Hospital, Boston Women's Lying-in, the Massachusetts College of Pharmacy and, finally, the old red-brick building with the four white pillars in front that was Angell Memorial Animal Hospital.

Since it was Saturday, we found a parking space right in front of the hospital. There were two doors. The one to the right was for clients and patients, the one to the left, for staff. Between them was an archway, with huge gates, that spanned a cobblestone driveway. Emily told me the entrance was previously used for large animals. It led to an enormous courtyard where they used to treat cows and horses. My blood raced as we mounted the steps to the staff doorway. I could already picture myself wearing hospital greens, a stethoscope draped casually around my neck.

Once inside, we climbed the black steel staircase to the second floor, our footsteps clanging through the dimly lit stairwell, until we reached the brick colonnaded walkway overlooking the courtyard. Emily explained that the building was exactly as it was when it was built in the early 1900s. It had never been modernized. The aura of Victorian must hanging over it was completely authentic. Off of the colonnade were the ten patient wards, ICU and surgery. The wards were brightly lit. There were separate ones for dogs, cats and exotics, each with clean and roomy cages. Surgery looked like nothing I knew at Dr. Waters's. There were six operating tables in a large, white-tiled room that gleamed with the kind of hygienic efficiency I had seen only in the movies. As we stood peeking through the heavy double doors that led to the surgery, two young doctors wearing real hospital greens pushed by us with a sedated dog on a rolling stretcher. At that moment, they were the embodiment of everything I ever wanted to be. They were followed by an older man, also wearing greens, who did a double take when he saw Dr. Addison.

"Emily, is that you? What the hell are you doing here? I thought you were down in Washington." He grabbed both her hands and smiled broadly. "I used to keep pretty good tabs on you."

"Hello, Jack," she said quietly, seeming to pull back a bit. "I've been up here almost a year. Got tired of all that big city high life. You remember, I'm just a country girl at heart. I'm with a small practice in Concord, now. I've just brought our future colleague here in for a quick Cook's tour. Do you mind?" She disengaged her hands from his and introduced me to Dr. Jack Richardson, Chief of Surgery, a tall man with graying sideburns and a fierce mustache. His voice was a deep baritone, like a radio announcer's.

"Mind? Hell no, I'm delighted. But why didn't you call me? Let me know you were back in town?" He turned to me, put his hand on my shoulder and spoke confidentially, "Did you know Dr. Addison was one of the brightest interns we ever had at Angell? If she'd listened to me and stayed and taken her boards in surgery, she'd be on staff right now." He paused. "It's not too late, Emily, you can still do that if you want to—but I suppose you're still into all that flying stuff."

Emily's face reddened. I saw a flash of anger in her eyes. "I made my choice a long time ago, Jack. I'll stand by it." She fussed with the catch on her shoulder-strap purse and shifted her weight impatiently from one foot to the other. "Well, it was nice to see you again. I want to show Steve some more of the hospital now, because we have to get back to Concord."

Her abruptness didn't put him off. "Oh, Emily," he persisted, "don't go running away again. Why don't you finish your tour with Steve and then have a cup of coffee with me? I've got a splenectomy to do, take me about an hour, then I'm free. Come on, Emily, I want to talk to you, know how you are. After all, it's been twelve years!"

I desperately wanted Emily to say yes. Coffee with the Chief of Surgery was much more than I had hoped for. But I could see from the expression on her face, it wasn't going to be.

"Thanks, Jack, we can't. Steve has to get home."

I almost blurted, No, I don't. I can stay as long as you like— But Emily's blue eyes turned almost gray, warning me to say nothing.

"OK," Richardson relented, "but you're not so far away now.

Why don't you call me and we'll have lunch, if only for old times' sake?"

"I will, Jack." Emily extended her hand. He held it a beat too long.

"Good-bye, Steve, I'll be looking for you," he said to me and pushed through the double doors into surgery.

The chance meeting with Jack Richardson blackened Emily's mood. She walked so quickly down the hospital corridor, I had to run to keep up with her. "That man's incredible; he's completely rewritten history." She was talking to herself, not to me. "How dare he say *he* wanted me to stay and take my boards. Do you know—" She turned to me finally in frustration. "Do you know, when he found out I was seeing Thom, he ran me ragged, made my life a living hell. I was interested in a surgical specialty then. Jack was already on staff and he was my supervisor, but how bright I was, or how good a vet I was, didn't interest him. I was a woman, and as far as he was concerned, a woman had only one purpose. When Thom came into the picture, he realized that was impossible, although it would've been impossible even if Thom hadn't been there, so he really turned on me. Just thinking about it makes me livid!" she sputtered. "*He* wanted me to take my boards! He wanted another girl friend, not another veterinary surgeon!"

Back in the forties and fifties when Dr. Addison was at vet school and interning at Angell, women were a rarity in the profession. There was an unwritten law that no more than two women would be accepted in any class in any recognized veterinary school. They were tokens and they had to be brilliant tokens, at that. For a woman to become a vet, she had not only to love animals, but to be an academic crackerjack, in some cases to the exclusion of everything else in her life. Then when she finally made it out into the real world of veterinary practice, unless she was liberated enough, ambitious enough and financially stable enough to set up her own practice, she often had to suffer the indignity of working for a man not nearly her professional equal, at wages he wouldn't dare to offer someone of his own sex. The course of study for a would-be veterinarian, male or female, was certainly arduous enough, without the added burden of exploitive and bigoted attitudes on the part of the veterinary establishment. Happily, in the sixties and early seventies, with the passage of the Equal Opportunity acts and the Bakke decision, the situation changed radically. Now, women comprise about 40 percent of every vet-school class, and their numbers are growing so rapidly they may soon be the majority in the profession. Unfortunately, all of that came too late for Emily Addison.

To my knowledge, she never did call Dr. Richardson. That was the last time either of us saw him. He left Angell Memorial in 1973, the year before I began my internship.

The Piper Cub circled the small airstrip at Concord. Emily lowered the flaps and nosed into the wind. "Steve, I'm leaving Dr. Waters at the end of the month." She didn't look at me. Instead, she kept her eyes on the small landing strip ahead. My heart sank. What I had long feared was finally going to happen. So much for my pull with God. "I've been offered a position in a practice in San Diego and I've decided to take it."

"San Diego," I moaned. "That's so far away, I'll never see you again." I slid down in my seat as far as the seat belt would allow. In that moment, my world had collapsed.

She gently set the plane down and rolled it to a stop near the hangar. "Of course you'll see me again. I'm a flyer, remember. I'll be back for a visit. Or maybe, when I'm settled, you'll come out and spend some time with me during the summer." She took off her dark glasses, turned to me and raised my chin from my chest, where it had fallen. "We've been good friends, Steve, and we'll stay good friends. I'm not going to die. I'm not even going to China. San Diego isn't the end of the earth. I'll write to you often, and you can write to me how things are with old Scrooge Waters."

"If you're not there, there's no reason for me to be there. I'll quit," I sulked.

"No you won't. You'll stay and learn as much as you can, even from Waters. You'll go to vet school and then you'll go on to Angell. I plan to write your recommendation myself. So let's hear no more about quitting. You're a special boy, Steve. You care so much about animals and you have a great talent for handling them. It would be a shame if all that went to waste."

Three weeks later, she was gone. I wrote to her three or four times a week in the beginning, and she answered back. Then our letters tapered off and finally, after a year or so, stopped. I was to see Emily again, but that would be eight years later.

Chapter 4

She was a tiny woman and she carried a cane with a silver handle in the shape of a dog. When I had first met her several years ago, the cane was only for effect, but now she needed it. She sat on the hard wooden bench outside the treatment booths, her thin, bony hands clutching the silver handle so tightly her knuckles were white. Mrs. Benson had always been delicate, but she seemed to have become even more frail since I last saw her two nights before. She was very pale, and her skin had a stretched, translucent quality, with a color that bordered on jaundice. The usual twinkle was gone from her soft brown eyes. She looked fatigued and worn, and for the only time in the two years I'd known her, she seemed really old. Every one of her seventy-five years was clearly reflected in her deeply lined face.

Even so, there was the aura of something very special about her that set her above and apart from the noise and hubbub of the people and animals in the hospital corridor. She had a presence, and even though she was small, when she entered a room she filled it. Mrs. Benson had been a theatrical costume designer, and her flair for clothes was still evident in the black cloak she wore tonight, fastened at the neck with a silver chain. Her husband, before he died, was a curator of eighteenth-century paintings at the Metropolitan Museum, and from the stories she'd told me, I gathered they knew everyone there was to know in New York in the thirties and forties. Now that he was gone, she lived alone with her cat, Eloise, in a tiny apartment, somehow managing to survive the daily battles of life on the Upper West Side.

Seated next to her was a gray-haired man of about sixty with an extravagant walrus mustache like Teddy Roosevelt's. He was as rotund and robust as she was thin and pale. He kept his hand at her elbow in a courtly manner, as if they were crossing a street. He was Mr. Robinson, her neighbor.

The very nature of night emergency service makes it difficult to develop personal relationships with clients. It's usually just in and out. I treat the animal, then turn it and its owner over to day-shift medical or surgical services. But there are those who over the years have become regulars, either because they haven't the time to take their animal to a vet during the day or simply because they liked me. Mrs. Benson was one of the latter. From the first moment she stepped into my treatment booth with her cat, we had an immediate rapport. I was fascinated by what she was and by what she had been. It amused her to say that she had adopted me, but I think it was quite the reverse.

I knew she lived alone, and if I didn't hear from her for a month or so, I'd make it my business to call and check, just to see if she was all right. No matter what time of day or night I phoned, her response was always the same. "I was just thinking about you," she'd say. "Another minute, I'd have dialed your number."

I envisioned her sitting by the phone waiting, with a little comic-strip balloon over her head and me in it. It became a joke with us, and soon when I'd call, before she even had a chance to chirp her bright Hello, I'd say, "I know; you were just thinking about me." Mrs. Benson would giggle, pleased that I knew her well enough to catch her mannerisms.

Since she lived only three blocks from my apartment, sometimes I would drop by to give Eloise a vaccination or to clean her ears. It saved Mrs. Benson the trip across town to the AMC, and it gave me the opportunity to chat with her and to again inspect the walls of her small apartment, which were covered with framed photographs of famous actors, writers, artists and musicians, all inscribed to Carla—that was her first name—or to her husband, Will.

Noel Coward, Gertrude Lawrence, Helen Hayes and Cole Porter peered out at me, wearing bathing suits and summer flannels.

Mary Martin was astride a horse on some ranch and Dorothy Parker was on a white chaise under a palm tree. Some faces I didn't recognize, and she'd say, "Oh my dear, that's Katharine Cornell. You would have loved her, she had King Charles spaniels" or "That's John Steinbeck. He had a standard poodle. Went everywhere with him, you know." For my benefit, she always related the legends on the wall to their animals, in case I couldn't otherwise appreciate them.

Mrs. Benson was a sprite, and I treasured the time I spent with her. But lately, the nights at the hospital had been frantic and my days were equally busy. Though I thought about her, I hadn't called her and I suddenly realized I hadn't heard from her since before the summer. When I finally did phone last week, I knew immediately from the tone of her voice that something was very wrong. "I'm afraid Eloise and I aren't feeling very well," she said, without any of our usual banter.

"Do you feel well enough to bring her to the hospital or would you like me to come and see you?" I asked.

"No, I'm all right now. I think you'll probably need to make tests, so I'll bring her to you," she said with resignation.

She was waiting for me when I came on duty early Monday evening, the pallor of illness etched in her face. Trying not to betray how startled I was at her appearance, I led her into the treatment booth. The moment she took the cat out of the carrier, I knew it was bad news. If it was possible, the cat looked much worse than Mrs. Benson did.

Eloise was a big black domestic shorthair, with unusually large yellow eyes. She was playful and affectionate, with the friendly, lumpy personality of a dog. You could do anything with her, turn her upside down, throw her in the air, rough her up. Whatever attention she received elicited deep contented purrs. According to Mrs. Benson, she particularly enjoyed having someone read aloud to her, and when I'd last visited them, they were thoroughly engrossed in *A Tale of Two Cities*, not Eloise's favorite, her owner explained, because there was no part in it for a cat.

Mrs. Benson brushed Eloise constantly, so her coat was always lustrous and gleaming. Around her neck, she wore a yellow leather collar with bells on it that jangled when she moved. "So she can't surprise me," Mrs. Benson would say.

But this night her coat was dull and lifeless, and the collar, though fastened on the tightest hole, hung loosely around her throat. She was listless and badly dehydrated. When I pulled the skin away from her thin neck, there was no resiliency. I stood her up on the examining table, leaning her against my body for support. "That's a good girl, Eloise. Try and stand up just for a minute. You know I won't hurt you," I said to soothe her as I palpated her abdomen. Her kidneys were huge and nodular and her liver was much larger than it should have been. Her breathing was raspy and labored, and when I put my stethoscope to her, I heard muffled heart sounds and what I was certain was fluid in her chest. When I had finished, the cat sank back down on the table like a balloon when the air is let out.

Mrs. Benson had been watching me intently as I did the examination, trying to read my face for a hopeful sign. Unfortunately, I couldn't give her one. Eloise, I thought, had all the symptoms of advanced cancer. Oh, God, why did you wait so damned long to bring her in? I wanted to ask Mrs. Benson, but I didn't. There was no need to add guilt to the pain she was already feeling.

But she knew what I was thinking and bit her lower lip. "I know," she sighed heavily. "I should've brought her in sooner, but I've been sick myself." She leaned the cane against the exam table and stroked the cat's head with both hands. "I had a mastectomy last month and I've been going down the street to Sloan–Kettering for chemotherapy."

I felt my stomach flip when she said that. "Why didn't you call me? I thought we were friends."

"We are, Steve. You know how much I think of you. But you're so busy, you have your own life. I didn't want to bother you with my troubles." She didn't look up. She just kept stroking the cat's head as she spoke. "Mr. Robinson, my neighbor, took care of her while I was in the hospital and he wanted to call you, but I told him not to. I knew it was something bad and I was afraid she'd die in here without me. Then when I came home I waited because I knew she was really sick and I didn't want to lose her. Not yet. I just couldn't face it. She's only seven, you know."

I did know. I knew all about it. But I wished at that moment that I didn't know Carla Benson. That she was just another client who had come in off the street with a sick cat. But she wasn't, and now I would have to tell her that the creature she loved most in the world was suffering from the same disease that had attacked her and, if I had read the signs correctly, in all probability, would have to be put to sleep. In any case that's not easy to tell someone. But the problem was compounded with Mrs. Benson, first, because she was a friend and, second, because she was so sick herself. I feared that if she lost Eloise she might give up all hope for her own recovery. I had seen that happen several times before with older people who lived alone and maintained their connection with the world through a pet. The animal was a lifeline—something to care for, something to care about—if it died, they soon followed. I didn't want that to happen to Mrs. Benson.

I drew some blood from Eloise's leg and put it in a glass vial. The lab was still open, so the blood work could be done tonight, saving time for the oncology service when they took over the case in the morning. Though from the look of the cat, I doubted there was much they could do to help. The AMC is the only major animal hospital with a cancer clinic, and miraculous work is being done. But as with cancer in humans, miracles can happen only if it's caught in time.

Eloise mewed softly, and when I rubbed the cat behind the ears to comfort her, Mrs. Benson put her hand over mine, her eyes brimming with tears. "She's very bad, isn't she, Steve?"

"I'm afraid she's not good," I answered truthfully. "I think she has a form of cancer. I can't be certain how far it's gone until we get the blood work back, take some X rays and oncology looks at her tomorrow." I was hedging a little, buying another day of hope for her. Maybe that wasn't the right thing to do, but I couldn't bring myself to tell her flat out what I really thought.

"If it is cancer, can't they do chemotherapy, like I've been having? It seems to be working." The last words caught in her throat. Her face was contorted with tears, no longer controlled, and her frail shoulders heaved with sobs. I put my arms around her, trying to comfort her as best I could.

"I'll see to it that everything humanly possible is done for Eloise. You know that, don't you?" I raised her chin with my hand, so that she could see that I meant it. Carla Benson sniffled like a little girl. She reached in her purse and pulled out a neatly pressed handkerchief.

"You must think I'm a silly old woman to love this cat so much," she said, dabbing at her eyes. "I'm sorry, I just can't help it. She's all I've got."

She pulled herself away from me and went back to the exam table. She picked the cat up in her arms and cradled it against her face, her hand gently caressing the soft black ears. They flicked at her touch and, sick as she was, Eloise closed her eyes and purred. "When Will died five years ago, I thought I wanted to die too. Then this wonderful black ball of fluff came into my life. She gave me so much and asked for so little in return—how could I not love her?" She began to cry again.

I unbuckled the collar from around the cat's neck and took her from Mrs. Benson's arms. "We're going to do our best for her," I promised. "Try not to worry. I'll call you the minute I know something." I gave her the collar, which she carefully put in her purse.

Still holding Eloise, I picked up Mrs. Benson's cane and handed it to her, and with my arm around her shoulders, led her out into the corridor. "Can you get a cab OK? Or do you want to wait here for a minute and I'll take you downstairs as soon as I take Eloise back to ICU?"

"No need for that." She took a deep breath and stood up a little straighter. "I'll be fine. It's still light out. I can get a cab at the entrance." She turned to the cat and brushed the top of its head with her lips. Then she took my hand and pressed it tightly. "Thank you for being so kind to both of us. I appreciate it, Steve."

"Promise me you won't worry too much. You need to take good care of yourself. I'll take care of Eloise."

"I promise." She pressed her lips together to avoid more tears and walked slowly down the corridor toward the exit, looking small and very vulnerable, her cane tapping lightly at her side. But her theatricality was still there. She knew I was watching and, without turning or looking back, she raised her hand and waggled her fingers in a good-bye gesture.

When Mrs. Benson had gone, I took Eloise back to ICU, where she would remain until oncology picked her up. Coincidentally, John Isaacs was sitting on the exam table talking to Penny Soames. John was a resident in oncology and was planning to make this his specialty. He was particularly fond of Penny, and when he had any free time, he liked to come down to ICU and gossip with her. About thirty-five, he was tall and skinny, with longish dark hair and a black beard. He looked like someone who might have sat at the table with Jesus.

"Hey Stevo, watchya got there?" he said when he saw me come in. "Doesn't look too good."

"She's gonna be in your bailiwick tomorrow. She's kind of a special case. Belongs to a friend of mine. Want to take a look?" John jumped off the table, and I put Eloise in his place.

"I got in under the wire at the lab, so you'll have the blood work first thing in the morning," I told him. He was palpating the cat's abdomen.

"Kidney's nodular, liver's enlarged," he said as his fingers worked the cat's belly and moved up to the glands around her neck.

"Yeah, and there's some fluid in her chest. I've asked for chest and abdominal rads."

John put his stethoscope to the cat's chest to hear for himself. "Yeah, you're right," he said after a minute. "Doesn't look promising, but we'll see what the bloods say. Who does she belong to?"

I told him about Mrs. Benson, and he nodded sympathetically when I explained how ill she was herself. "If there's anything you guys can do, anything at all, do it!"

"I'll look out for her, but don't be too hopeful." He was being honest. I don't know what else I expected him to say. I could see the cat's condition for myself. I guess even I wanted some kind of miracle.

Penny, who had finished putting a beagle with a collapsed trachea in the oxygen unit, came over to the table and looked at Eloise. "What do you think's wrong?" she asked.

"Probably lymphoma or lymphosarcoma," John answered matter-of-factly.

"Poor baby," she clucked, petting Eloise's head.

"Yeah, and she's got some breathing problems," I said. "So I'd like you to keep an eye on her tonight."

"I don't think there's any room; we're all full up." She gestured at the cages. Every one was occupied. I went from cage to cage, looking to arrange a vacancy by moving an animal who was well enough not to need ICU's constant attention. As I walked down the line, those who could barked and meowed for my attention. Others lay quietly in their cages, too sick to make any kind of fuss.

We couldn't move the post-op Siamese, nor the epileptic Chihuahua and certainly not the Doberman HBC. But in the last cage on the upper level, a small brown and white terrier mix with one ear up and one ear down cocked his head and looked at me alertly when I peered in the cage. I glanced at the chart on the cage door—three fractured ribs and a pneumothorax.

"How about this guy? He's looking pretty perky." I opened the door and patted the dog on the head.

"That's Toby. He's a 'drop-off,' " Penny said over my shoulder. "Some son of a bitch kicked him in the chest and then abandoned him. A neighbor brought him in, but can't keep him. Gotta find a home for him."

I put my stethoscope to Toby's chest. His lungs sounded clear. "You're doin' real good, fella. What say we move you to a ward and give old Eloise your spot?" Toby cocked his head again as if he understood every word I had said. I carefully lifted him out of the cage, gave him to Penny and replaced him with the cat. Penny took the dog down the hall to the ward where he would stay until he had fully recovered. Meanwhile, she would spread the word in the animal-lover's underground that a home was needed for him. In Toby's case, that probably wouldn't be too difficult. He was young and a dead ringer for that movie dog, Benji. Penny wouldn't have to use hard sell on this one.

I glanced at Eloise lying on her side in the cage, depressed and very sick. Until the diagnosis was confirmed, there was no point in making her more uncomfortable with any kind of treatment. If John and I were right, no treatment would be possible. Once again, I was helpless. Damn it! I hated that feeling. I kicked my foot against the treatment table John Isaacs was sitting on. "How do you do it? How can you bear it?" I asked him. "I get two or three cancer cases a week and that's too many. How can you possibly see this kind of thing ten hours a day every day of the week and not go nuts?"

"I don't know. Sometimes I wonder how much longer I *can* take it." He swung around on the table so that he faced me. "You know Sara Davidson is leaving the unit. This morning she said to me, 'God, they're all dying, and the clients are always crying and so upset. I can't bear it another minute.' So she's quitting for private practice. I was in private practice for five years. You know what that is—ear infections, vaccinations, fleas. It gets goddamned boring." He pulled on his beard and thought for a moment. "I wanted to make some sort of contribution—to medicine, maybe to life. So when the residency in oncology opened up here, I grabbed it. But it gets to you. Cancer is scary enough when it happens to human beings, but at least people can accept the responsibility for their own life-style. They drank too much, they smoked too much, they worked in the wrong factory and inhaled asbestos or coal dust. But when it happens to their innocent animals, they just can't understand it. They feel responsible: 'Why my dog?' 'Why my cat?' And before you know it, they're carrying suitcases filled with guilt. They didn't feed the animal right, they didn't care for it properly, they didn't see the symptoms soon enough. They're devastated, and it's tough to handle, because you not only have to be a good veterinarian, you have to be a chemotherapist and a psychiatrist as well. You don't just take care of the animals, you take care of the whole family. And there you are—the dog is crying, the people are crying and you're crying right along with them. Sometimes it gets so intense I think my head's gonna blow off. Terminal illness is shit! I don't have to tell you that. But there are those cases where the surgery works, or the chemotherapy works, or maybe God works—who knows? But there's the dog or the cat running around two years after the cancer was diagnosed. For me, that's what it's all about. Besides, we've got the new immunotherapy thing going with breast cancer in dogs, and the people at Sloan–Kettering are real excited. They think it may have great possibilities for people."

John was all wound up. As he spoke, the excitement shone in his dark eyes and I understood why. Even so, I knew I couldn't last ten minutes in the oncology unit. The cure ratio was just too low and the pain ratio, for both animals and humans, too high. The daily drama of night emergency was bad enough.

John read my face. "It's not all tears, you know. Sometimes we get a laugh or two. Like the guy who thought his dog, Zero, would get nauseated from chemotherapy. Well dogs don't, you know, and they don't lose their hair either. But this fellow was sure his dog would. So every week after he brought the dog in for treatment, he'd buy a whole bunch of pot, and he and Zero, this big shaggy, mixed breed, would go home and he'd blow the grass in the dog's face so he wouldn't be nauseated, and they'd both get all tore up." John chuckled at the thought of the incongruous stoned pair. "Well, this went on for a whole year, and finally last week we had to put the dog to sleep, so the guy brought in his whole stash of pot and gave it to the oncology unit as a gift. Friday night we got all tore up in Zero's honor and had a terrific time." He jumped down off the table, and his wooden-soled clogs clattered when they hit the floor. "See, it isn't all bad, Stevo," he said, smiling wryly.

Two days later, he called me to confirm our earlier diagnosis. Eloise had advanced lymphosarcoma and the cancer had spread too far for any kind of therapy. She would have to be put to sleep.

Mrs. Benson's hand shook as I led her into the treatment booth. Tyler, the clinic aide, had brought Eloise in from the ward and placed her on the exam table. She looked even more debilitated than she had on Monday, and Mrs. Benson sucked in her breath when she saw her.

"Are you sure you want to do it this way?" I asked her.

"I'll hold her for you, if you like," Mr. Robinson, her neighbor, offered. He had accompanied us into the booth, continuing to keep his hand at her elbow for support.

"No," she answered firmly, "it's my place to hold her, no one else's."

I prepared two syringes, one with sodium pentothal, a barbiturate, and the other with a solution we call "The Kiss of Death," T-61. It's the latter that does the job. But sometimes, though the animal feels no pain, T-61 causes extreme muscle twitching, a really rotten thing for an owner to see. It's hard enough to watch something you love die, without the added unpleasantness of rigors and spasms. So if there's going to be a witness, I prefer to use the pentothal first.

But no matter what kind of fancy, velvet-lined box I put it in to soothe my psyche, I hate putting animals to sleep. For me, it's one of the more onerous things about being a veterinarian. It's always been difficult, and if I practiced for the next fifty years, it would never be easy—even when I know, as now with Eloise, that there's no other merciful course of treatment possible. Each time, a great mix of thoughts and feelings flash through my mind, eventually settling in the pit of my stomach like a rusty cannonball. It has to do with the knowledge that I have the power to snuff a life in seconds—just like that—and the dreadful emotional wrench I know the loss will cause the people connected to that small life, Carla Benson for instance. Yet I do it every night, sometimes two or three times in the same night.

Of course, I can take solace in the fact that I can do legally what no M.D. can do: I can put an end to suffering for a living creature. Small comfort that is. But after seven years of practice, I've found a way to let a kind of psychic shield clang down around my heart. If I didn't, I'd be a likely candidate for a shrink. I could only hope that trusty shield would be there now when I desperately needed it.

Carla Benson was leaning heavily on her cane when I gave her the hospital's standard euthanasia release form to sign. She laid the cane against the wall and, using the exam table for support, scratched her name at the bottom of the page without reading it.

"Would you like a chair? Do you want to sit down?" I offered.

"No need for that. I'm all right as I am," she answered with determination. "Just put her in my arms. I want to hold her for just a little bit."

I lifted Eloise off the table and gently placed her in Mrs. Benson's outstretched hands. She pressed the small black form to her chest and rocked the badly emaciated cat like a baby. "My poor little friend, how I will miss you," she whispered hoarsely, rubbing her face against Eloise's ears. "But you're so sick, and this will be better for both of us. It *is* better, don't you think, Robbie?" She turned to Mr. Robinson, who now seemed even more upset than she was. A tear trickled down his ruddy face, and rather than speak, he put his hand on her arm and nodded.

"It's the kindest thing we can do," I answered for him. "If we let her go on, there'll be pain, and I know you don't want that for her."

"No, of course not. I just wanted to keep her with me as long as possible. She's such a funny, silly little cat. She always made me laugh so. Eloise never had a proper sense of decorum and no idea that cats are supposed to be aloof and independent. She followed me around all day. From the moment she woke me with her sandpaper tongue in the morning until I turned out the light at night, she was at my side. The apartment is so empty now. I don't know if I can bear it without her. Who will I read to?" She pulled the cat closer and rocked her harder. "But I don't want her to suffer, not for a minute."

"She won't, I promise." I held the pentothal syringe up for her to see. "This is an anesthetic. She'll just close her eyes and go to sleep."

"Did you hear that, my little darling? It's going to be OK. It won't hurt you at all." The tears had started in Mrs. Benson's eyes and they tumbled down her cheeks onto the cat's fur.

Ordinarily, I would have had a clinic aide hold the animal

steady while I administered the solution. But there was no need for that in this case. The cat barely moved. Both Mrs. Benson and Mr. Robinson averted their eyes as I held Eloise's left foreleg and injected the anesthetic into a vein. Within seconds, she had gone limp in Mrs. Benson's arms. I quickly injected the T-61, and by the time I slowly and silently counted to five, it had reached her heart. Eloise was dead.

Mrs. Benson seemed stunned. She was oblivious to the noisy cacophony of animal life that floated through the closed door from the corridor and waiting room. I took the cat from her arms and gave it to Tyler, who had waited outside. He would take the body back to a holding room until Mrs. Benson decided what she wanted done with it.

Mr. Robinson recovered himself and led her to the steel folding chair in the corner of the booth. She collapsed on it, her head in her hands. I tried very hard to think this was just another cat I had put to sleep, but it wasn't. My stomach was in a knot, my head ached and I was fighting back my own tears. My famous shield seemed to have deserted me. I put my hand on Mrs. Benson's thin shoulder, "Can I get you anything? Would you like some water?"

She reached back and patted me comfortingly. "No, dear, nothing. I'll be all right in a minute. I didn't mean to go all queasy on you. I just had no idea it would be so fast. One minute she was there and the next—gone. Where to, I wonder? I'd like to think that odd little soul is waiting for me somewhere. Do you suppose she is, Steve?" She looked up at me like a child wanting to be told there are angels in heaven.

"Maybe she is. Maybe they all are. All the dogs and cats we've ever loved." Why not? It was a reassuring thought and perhaps it would help get her through the next few lonely days. Who knows? Maybe it was true.

I hated to bring this up now. It was sticky and insensitive, but it was hospital policy and I had to. People were funny about the disposition of their pets. Some had them put to sleep and then just walked out the door, leaving the means of disposal to us. But others, as if it were a close relative, were very particular about how it was done, either wanting the body donated to the hospital for necropsy, or cremated so they could scatter the remains where the pet was happiest. Some took the body with them and arranged elaborate funerals at pet cemeteries. In any event, I had to ask. "What would you like us to do with Eloise?" I stammered. "We can handle everything if you like, or would you prefer to have her cremated and have her ashes?"

Mrs. Benson was surprisingly calm and forthright. "I'd like her cremated, Steve. Then I can scatter her ashes in the garden below us. She sat in the window by the hour and stared at that garden. I think if Eloise had any secret wish it was to jump out and play in it."

Mr. Robinson spoke up gruffly. "Considering you live on the tenth floor, Carla, I'd say it was a good thing she didn't."

"Well, she'll be in it now and that'll be a good thing too." Mrs. Benson smiled for the first time. "Will you see to it, Steve?"

"I'll take care of everything. You go home and try to get a good night's sleep. I'll bring you the ashes in a day or so. Then—" I hesitated for a minute. "Then next week we'll talk about a new kitten."

Mrs. Benson was shocked. "Oh, Steve, I couldn't. Not now. Eloise is barely gone, and besides, I'm too old and too sick to begin again with a new one."

"That's rubbish!" Mr. Robinson said flatly. "Be the best thing in the world for you. What's more, you've got a built-in baby-sitter—me!" He pounded his chest with his fist.

Maybe I should have given her more time to accept Eloise's death, but to be honest, I didn't feel there was time to play with. She needed another animal and she needed one quickly. If I just planted the seed tonight, she could mull it over for a few days, and with the feisty Mr. Robinson as my ally, maybe she'd relent. At least it was worth a try.

Her black cape wrapped around her like a blanket, she rose from the chair with some effort. Mr. Robinson sprang to her side to assist her, handing her the cane. She leaned on it and looked up at me, her eyes still reddened from tears. "I know you both mean well, but it's too hard. I don't think I could go through it again," she sighed. "You learn to love these little things, they become the center of your life and a part of your being. Then they're taken away from you. It's not fair. I should be old enough to know that few things in life are fair. But I'm certain, when I close my eyes for the last time, I'll still be saying, 'It's not fair.' I simply haven't the strength to get involved another time." She took my hand and held it firmly. "Thank you, Steve, for being so kind and thank you for caring. I hope you'll come by and have tea with me even though Eloise is gone?"

"You know I will. It was always you I came to see. Eloise was just a good excuse." I leaned down and kissed her on the cheek, trying hard not to betray the lump that had been in my throat for the past ten minutes.

Mr. Robinson shook my hand, and they were gone, disappearing into the sea of people and animals in the waiting room. I closed the booth door tightly and sagged against it. The tears I had been holding back finally were free. I didn't want anyone to see me.

Chapter 5

"DOCTOR KRITSICK, EMERGENCY BOOTH 7! DOCTOR KRITSICK EMERGENCY BOOTH 7, PUL-EAZE!"

Carmen's voice on the loudspeaker rudely intruded on my daydream abruptly bringing me back to the din of the Animal Medical Center. I hurried down the corridor to Booth 7, and Jim Hartley, a first-year intern, met me at the door. He was nervous and badly flustered, "I've got a scalded puppy. Thought you should have a look before I began treatment."

What Hartley really meant was he didn't know what to do. Scalded puppies aren't in the regular curriculum in vet school. This one lay collapsed and quivering in a towel on the exam table. She was tiny, no more than eight weeks old, with the soft not quite formed features of all babies, animal or human. Her black hair was still wet, and she squealed when I parted it to look at the angrily inflamed skin beneath. Blisters were beginning to form on her ears and abdomen and the skin on her nose was raw. Her owner, a thin, wiry Hispanic man with a pockmarked face, hovered over the table.

"What happened? Tell me quickly!" I snapped at him.

"I donno, Doc. I donno how it happened. My kid, she was gonna give the dog a bath, I think. I donno what she done. She only eight. I hear the dog yell. I run into the bathroom. The kid have only hot water in the tub. I grab the dog an' bring it here. It gonna be OK, you think? I pay whatever you want!"

Now he wants to pay. Now, when it's probably too late. How could he let the kid do that? Doesn't anyone watch? Doesn't anyone ever pay attention? Doesn't he know an eight-week-old puppy shouldn't have a bath in the first place? Of course he doesn't know. He can barely take care of himself and his kid, much less a dog. Sometimes the stupidity and irresponsibility I see in people here makes me want to punch my fist through a wall!

"The puppy is in shock," I told him. "She's been badly burned over her whole body. I honestly don't know if she'll make it, but we'll try." I turned to the intern. "Hartley, let's get her back to ICU and get fluids into her as quickly as possible."

I gently lifted the small, whimpering mass of wet black fur off the table and wrapped her in the towel. "We're gonna make you feel better, baby. It'll be all right," I whispered to her.

"You fix it up, Doc, I pay you anything. Anything!"

"Yeah, sure," I said over my shoulder and ran down the corridor to ICU. Hartley fluttered behind me, his wooden clogs, a symbol of "cool" for interns at the AMC, clattering on the linoleum-tile floor. Hartley was anything but cool. He should've known what to do. Scalding is no different from any other burn case. It's emergency medicine and the essence of emergency medicine for animals as well as humans, is time. Minutes, even seconds, count. This baby should've had fluids in her ten minutes ago. I was annoyed with Hartley's incompetence and wondered if he would ever learn. Night emergency at the AMC can be overwhelming, even for me, and I've been doing it for three years. For an intern fresh out of Colorado State University with only a few months in this animal Bellevue under his belt it can be staggering. Even so, I had my doubts about Jim Hartley.

"It's a scalding," I said to Penny Soames in ICU. "Looks like second- and third-degree burns over three-quarters of the body. We'll need IV fluids and steroids right away, she's real shocky. Let's use lactated Ringer's with 2½ percent dextrose added and 100 mg of Solu–Delta–Cortef."

Before the words were out of my mouth, she was rigging the IV fluids and inserting a jugular catheter in the puppy's throat. With a syringe, she quickly injected the steroids into the catheter's extension tube. Penny put her lips close to the small black head and murmured in its blistered ear, "It's OK now, little one.

It's OK. I'm gonna take care of you. How'd this ever happen to you, sweetheart?" She noted the raw and peeling skin on the nose and abdomen.

"Kid gave it a bath in scalding water," I answered for the puppy.

"Christ!" She grimaced with sympathetic pain. "I'd like to throw the whole family in scalding water! See how they like it!"

"Let's try and save this baby first," I said, and put a thermometer in the puppy's rectum.

"OK, Hartley." The intern was leaning over my shoulder. "What's next? The puppy is in shock, slightly dehydrated. The skin is peeling and inflamed and—" I looked at the thermometer, "the temperature is 99.5°." Normal for a dog is about 102°.

"We should apply topical cream for the burns and keep the patient warm," Hartley volunteered.

"You get the cigar," Penny muttered. He was not her favorite intern, and as far as practical knowledge was concerned, she had it all over him. She was already shaving the puppy down so that Sulfamyalon Cream could be rubbed on the badly burned skin.

"What about antibiotics, Hartley?" I asked.

"Yes, of course, antibiotics. That goes without saying."

"Nothing goes without saying." I was short with him. "In emergency medicine you have to be quick, but you must be thorough. With a burn case, after you've treated for shock you think about secondary infection." I prepared a syringe with Keflex, an antibiotic, and injected it into the catheter.

"Penny, when you finish rubbing the cream on, put her in a cage with some heat lamps. That's about all we can do for her now. I just hope she makes it through the night."

"She'll make it, I'll see to that!" Penny's dark brown eyes glinted with determination.

Hartley and I went back to the clinic booth to speak with the puppy's owner, Hector Arroyo. If she lived, the dog's treatment would be costly, since she'd have to be hospitalized for at least a week. However, if Arroyo was willing, the hospital would work out a payment schedule over a long period of time. But the booth was empty. There was no sign of Hector Arroyo in the hall or the reception area.

"Did you see where the guy in seven went?" I asked Carmen at the desk.

"Skinny guy, bad skin?"

"Yeah, we left him here about ten minutes ago."

"He's gone."

"Did he say he'd be back?" Hartley asked.

"No, he didn't say nothing. He just went."

"Damn it, Jim, that pup's a drop-off. Damn, Damn!" I kicked the front of the reception desk. I should've known. Usually, I can smell a drop-off coming, but I was so involved with the dog and treating it quickly, I didn't pay attention to the owner—not that I could've prevented his leaving.

"But he said he'd pay anything!" Hartley sounded personally wounded.

"Yeah, they always say that. 'Take care of my dog, Doc, I'll give you my wife, my car, the shirt off my back,' then they split! Christ, people make me sick. They hurt 'em then they dump 'em!"

I left Hartley in the night pharmacy to deal with the paperwork on the puppy. She had already been admitted to the hospital, so if she survived the night, she'd be treated and cared for until she was well. Her future was another matter.

A ruckus had started in the reception area and I went out to investigate. It seemed the sky had fallen. Henny-Penny, Chicken Little and Turkey-Lurkey were clustered around the desk, all talking at once. In the midst of it was Kenny Gilbert, the third intern on the night roster. Short and stocky, with a halo of Harpo Marx yellow, curly hair, Kenny had the look as well as the disposition of a precocious teenager. He'd arrived at the AMC at the same time as Jim Hartley, but unlike Hartley, he had quickly acclimated himself to the breakneck pace and within a matter of weeks was handling his cases with the deftness of someone with much more experience. In fact, he was the only new intern I didn't have to prod to work faster when the case load backed up.

From the first, he established himself as unofficial social director for interns and residents and the off-time parties he gave in the tiny closetlike apartment he maintained over a Chinese restaurant were musts on everyone's social calendar. Kenny loved the bizarre, and since bizarre was standard nightly fare, working night emergency was no chore for him.

"What's going on?" I asked Carmen.

"It's him, Doctor Kritsick. The man with the dog, who ain't got no dog." She nodded in the direction of a well-dressed, middle-aged man who was shouting at Gilbert. They were surrounded by what seemed to be every dog owner and dog in the crowded waiting room, all talking and barking at once.

"What do you mean, 'he ain't got no dog'?"

"Just what I said. He ain't got one and he says it's biting him," Carmen sighed. "It's full moon ya know."

I remembered Amelia's warning when I first came in tonight. This was one of her "crips." I pushed my way to the front of the desk, toward Gilbert.

"Ah, Doctor Kritsick, perhaps you can help." Kenny spoke as if I were Henry Kissinger just landed to negotiate the Arab-Israeli peace. "This gentleman is Mister Edelman. His dog is being attacked and bothered by the other dogs in the room and it's gotten so nervous, it's biting his leg." He formally introduced me to the besieged man.

"How do you do, Mister Edelman." I fully assumed the role of visiting diplomat, even to the point of a slight bow.

"Man, this guy's nuts," a black man the size of Mean Joe Greene shouted over the barks of the Doberman he held tightly by the collar. "He says my dog bit his dog and he's callin' the cops. This crazy ain't got no dog. Man, you should call the guys with the butterfly net, that's what you should do!"

"He grabbed Bitsy right out of my arms. Said he was taking her to a cage so his dog would be safe. We won't be safe till he's out of here!" The elderly gray-haired woman, clutching a pop-eyed, overweight Boston bull terrier, stamped her foot to make her point.

COMFORTS

"See? They're upsetting him again," Mr. Edelman wailed. "He's at my leg! For God's sake, help me get him off my leg! George, stop it! Down, I say!" He furiously brushed at his well-tailored trousers.

"What do you suggest we do, Doctor Kritsick?" Kenny Gilbert asked in his most professional tone.

"I'm not sure, Doctor Gilbert. It's the first time I've ever dealt with this breed."

"What do you mean, the first time you ever dealt with this breed!" Edelman shouted angrily. "What kind of vet are you? Haven't you ever seen a purebred fox terrier before?"

"Ah, a fox terrier. That's it, of course!" I had found the Rosetta stone. "They're very high strung, as you know, Doctor Gilbert. Perhaps if we gave him a tranquilizer it would quiet him down. What do you think?"

"Exactly right, Doctor Kritsick, and maybe I could find an extra lead for him. After all, Mister Edelman can't possibly control him without a lead."

"Good idea, Doctor Gilbert."

While Kenny went off to find a syringe and a lead, I shooed the gathered throng back to their seats in the waiting room. Mr. Edelman continued to slap at his leg.

"How long have you had George?" I asked out of real curiosity.

"He'll be three at Christmas. My wife gave him to me as a present." There was a tinge of sadness in his voice.

"Is she as attached to him as you are?" I was getting into the spirit of the thing.

"She was," he sighed, "but she's gone now."

"I'm sorry to hear that. When did you lose her?"

Edelman picked up a file folder from the desk and hit the side of his knee with it, "Down, boy, down! I didn't lose her, she left me. Thank God she didn't take George with her."

Kenny trotted up to the desk and handed me the syringe. He gave the lead to Edelman. "OK, Mister Edelman, Doctor Kritsick will give George the tranquilizer as soon as I attach the lead to his collar so you can hold him." Kenny knelt at Edelman's feet and fiddled in the air with the end of the lead. "Sit, George, sit! There's a good boy. All right, Doctor Kritsick. He's all yours. I'll keep him still for you."

I squatted next to Kenny and, with as much flair as I could muster, pushed the plunger on the empty syringe. "There, that should quiet him. This is Acepromazine, Mister Edelman, a pretty stiff dose. It may make him a bit wobbly, so I'd suggest carrying him home. But at least he'll sleep through the night."

Edelman wound the dangling lead around his wrist and, with a grunt, lifted the imaginary George in his arms. "What a relief! It's the first time in three hours he's been away from my leg. You guys are wonderful. What do I owe you?"

"There'll be no charge on this one," I said magnanimously. "George was never even in the treatment booth."

"Well, thanks. I'll bring him back if I have a problem."

"Yeah, you do that." Kenny tried hard to smother his giggles.

We watched Edelman as he walked through the waiting room, his empty arms out in front of him supporting the invisible sleeping dog. When he was through the double doors and safely out on the ramp, Kenny clutched his leg.

"Oh, Doctor! Help me! George is biting my leg! Down, boy! Down, I say!"

"Give him another shot of Ace."

"No, he'll O.D. Let's just lock him in, let someone else deal with him."

Kenny opened the sliding door to the clinic booth and pushed the imaginary dog inside, closing it behind him. "With any luck," he leered, "Hartley will be the next one in here."

It was the kind of lunatic camaraderie I had once shared with David. In funny ways, Kenny Gilbert reminded me of him.

Chapter 6

Not too long ago, my life was perfect, or at least I thought it was. There was no need to search for answers, since I had no questions. Everything had been clearly planned and mapped out for me since I was fourteen. But now, it was all a muddle. I no longer had a distinct vision of the years that lay before me. That naive, unthinking certainty that I would live forever, evaporated when David took ill. He was my best friend. The same age, we had grown up, played, laughed and gone to school together. We shared everything—secret thoughts, guilty consciences, dreams, even girls. Now, after an agonizing year, he was dead, and though I knew it was going to happen, the shock of the actual event left what felt like a cannonball-size hole in my chest that wouldn't go away. I missed him, of course. But along with that, my own mortality, something I'd never even considered before, was brought into question. Was I going the right way? Did this life I had chosen for myself have any meaning? More to the point, would I, unlike David, have the time to give it real purpose?

I hoped the answer would come to me as I ran the winding asphalt road between Lexington and Concord. Running helped me to think. It gave me a direct connection with the trees, the houses and the land I passed. It gave me a goal and somehow gave me flashes of great clarity. I'd been running ever since I hurt my knee playing touch football at Michigan State. A doctor there told me I could avoid surgery if I ran, because it would strengthen the muscles around the knee. So I ran. First two miles a day, then two and a half and soon, with ease, I doubled it to five. I ran all through the years at college and vet school. I even managed to

find time for an occasional run during the madness of interning at
Angell. When I returned to Lexington and began to run regularly, I upped the daily distance to ten miles.

I was keeping a good easy pace. The wind was behind me, and
the air was clear and crisp. It was a beautiful March morning.
Much more beautiful than it had any right to be, considering the
awful sadness I felt. If it had been cloudy and raining, it would've
better suited my mood. The sky and the earth should have been
crying for David, as I was. My destination was the Concord
Bridge, just over the town line from Lexington. I had been running the same route every morning, rain or shine, winter or summer, ever since I began working at George Carney's clinic almost
three years before. It seemed a lifetime ago.

George's clinic was housed in a handsome, one-story fieldstone
building he had designed himself. A pleasant place to work, it was
cheery, well-equipped and efficient. A sharp contrast to the urban
pressure-cooker atmosphere of the old, rundown Angell Memorial Animal Hospital in Boston. Carney's clientele was mostly affluent, well dressed, spoke English and usually paid their bills,
even if they crabbed about them. There were no cruelty cases, no
stabbings and the few gunshot wounds we treated were the result
of hunting accidents.

George Carney had built his practice from scratch and was
justly proud of it. He and his associate (that was me), dispensed
good veterinary care, his clients were happy, and most important
as far as he was concerned, he made a damned good living.
George wasn't interested in advancing academically in the profession. He didn't write scholarly articles for the journals and he
rarely read them. He kept up with progress in the field through
hearsay, and since I was hot off the academic griddle, he depended a good deal on me to keep him up to date through the
articles I read or the lectures I still attended at Angell. If a case
was too complicated or, occasionally, beyond our expertise, he
had sense enough to refer the patient to Angell for consultation.

Carney was an attractive, easy-going man of forty-five whose
life was completely circumscribed by his family. He allowed
nothing to interfere with the time he spent with his wife, Vicky,

and their three young daughters, especially not the clinic. Even emergencies were seen only during office hours. Not long after I entered his practice, he joined a pool of seventeen veterinarians in the area, formed to cover off-hour calls. That meant that once every seventeen days, our clinic was on duty after office hours. At any other irregular time, clients had to drive as much as forty-five minutes to have their animal seen, even if it was dying.

George had ample opportunity to expand the practice, to take on other associates, so that the clinic could remain open later in the evening and on weekends. I hated not seeing emergencies and volunteered to take that on. But George didn't want to set any precedents. He wasn't an overly ambitious vet. He was perfectly content with his life and his practice just as they were. My suggestions to the contrary, he had no intention of altering either.

When I first came to work for Carney, I had just finished my year of internship at Angell, perhaps the hardest, most grueling year of my life. I was exhausted, both physically and mentally, from the endless grind that combined treatment of cases with lectures and conferences, beginning at seven in the morning and ending well after midnight. Like so many other interns, while I was doing it, I hated it and wondered why I was putting myself through such systematic torture. But when it was over, I realized that I had learned more about veterinary medicine at Angell in one year than I might have in ten years of private practice. I had done well, and before graduation, I was offered a residency in surgery or internal medicine. As an intern, I had earned the munificent sum of $125 a week. By the time taxes and social security were taken from it, barely enough remained to buy my meals and put gas in the car. If I accepted the residency, I would be earning only slightly more.

At the same time, three jobs in private practices were dangled before me like tempting little cakes. The decision was a difficult one. As much as I wanted to stay at Angell and become board certified in a specialty, such as surgery, I felt the time had come for me to begin paying my own way and finally relieve my parents of the financial burden they had carried for twenty-three years. So private practice it was, and George Carney's offer proved to be the best of the three.

After the breakneck schedule of Angell, working for Carney was like being on a vacation. But I had to adjust to the slow, measured pace of a suburban animal clinic. There was actually time to talk with clients, to establish personal relationships with them and with their animals. There were free moments between appointments to laugh and socialize with other members of the staff. There weren't twenty cases backed up waiting to see me. I didn't have to fly off to a lecture. I didn't have to go without sleep to work a double shift. In effect, I had to get used to living like a normal person again.

In the beginning, when I first arrived at the clinic, I seemed to be moving double-time on a treadmill, while everyone around me was going in slow motion. How could they work that way, I wondered? How did they ever get anything done? Well, they did, I soon learned, and had a fine time doing it. It wasn't long before I was moving at their speed and thinking there never had been another.

Life couldn't have been sweeter. I had a job I liked, I was doing what I'd always dreamed of doing and at long last, I was financially independent. Since I was then making almost four times the salary I earned as an intern, I felt I finally could afford an apartment of my own and I quickly found a small studio in a singles complex in Arlington, about two miles from the clinic. I even had some money left at the end of the week—as well as the time and energy—to take a date to a proper dinner. During my internship, except when I had dinner with my parents, I had survived on a diet consisting mostly of pizza and Dunkin' Donuts, and any girl I took out didn't fare much better. But at twenty-three, I was on top of the world. To my way of thinking, I had everything. If there was a better way to live, I didn't yet know about it.

To add to my smug self-satisfaction, I had found a wonderful friend in Sabrina Metcalf, the clinic's receptionist-nurse, font of all information and gossip. Sabrina, not yet forty, was the mother of two teenage boys and recently divorced from her second husband. She was given to wearing peasant skirts and silver jewelry, a hangover from the years she lived in Big Sur with her first husband, a sculptor. She was warm, earthy and at times, terribly funny. I adored her on sight. She, in turn, immediately gathered me in and settled my place in her life as somewhere between a third son and a younger brother. I've always found it easy to relate to older women, and Sabrina was certainly no exception. It was she who helped me most when David became ill.

When I reached the Concord Bridge, I stopped to rest. It was still early—only 7:30. There was plenty of time before I had to start back to Lexington. I would shower and change in the bathroom at the clinic and, as usual, be ready for the first patient at nine. My body was tingling from the run. Perspiration ran down my face into the red bandana I had tied around my neck. I pressed my sweat shirt against my chest to absorb the moisture and zipped up the hooded jacket I wore over it. I had a navy wool watch cap pulled down over my ears, and lined leather gloves covered my hands. The air was cold, but I didn't feel the chill because the blood was racing so furiously through my veins. Usually, I didn't like to stop, especially if I had a good pace going and I wasn't tired. But this morning I needed more time before I once again began the daily routine that had become, over the last months, meaningless.

I leaned over the rail of the bridge and looked at the embankment below, the disputed site of the first Revolutionary battleground. There was great dissent between the residents of Lexington and Concord about which was really the first battleground, the Concord Bridge or the Lexington Green. I think it really was Lexington, and since I grew up there, I always owned on the side of the Green.

Large chunks of ice floated past in the stream beneath me, and the grass on the banks was a harsh, snow-bitten, winter brown. Even with the bright sun glinting on the water and the cloudless blue sky overhead, spring seemed an eternity away. This had been such a terribly cold winter, not just in terms of weather, which was certainly awful, but, as with David's illness, it seemed that whatever powers there were had conspired to make life for me relentlessly gray and grim. No longer could I skip along worrying only about my next date, or a new suit, or how I could con George into giving me a raise. This winter, finally, I learned about things outside of myself. I learned about pain, I learned about death and I learned that maybe, at last, it was time to grow up.

I noticed a single duck dodge a large piece of ice and make its way to the sparsely covered bank. Was it a lonely leftover, who had managed to survive the awful winter here in Concord, or had it just arrived from the south, a harbinger of spring? I watched it and thought about that day not quite a year ago when everything began to change, only I wasn't aware of it then. It was April, lovely and warm, the 27th of April, to be exact. I won't ever forget it. I was with a patient, and right after I finished, I planned to have lunch with David. We were going to talk about the shack at the Cape we had arranged to take for the summer, along with two other friends. The client, Mr. Kennedy, was a grumpy Yankee who required more bedside manner than his cat, Kato, one of my favorite patients.

I had just finished clipping Kato's claws, when Sabrina's voice crackled over the intercom in the treatment room.

"She's here again, Steve, and she'll only see you."

I held Kato in my arm and pushed the talk-back button with my free hand.

"Who's here?"

"Mrs. Wyman," Sabrina hissed. "The one with the mink coat and the malamute."

"Oh, God, no! Not her again!" The cat worked its way up my arm and settled itself comfortably around my neck. "Tell her I'm going into surgery right after I finish with this patient. Tell her I don't have time to see her, I have a lunch date. Tell her anything. Why can't George see her?" I was trying to whisper so that Mr. Kennedy wouldn't hear.

"You know she doesn't want George, she wants you. Besides, George went home early for lunch. Please see her, Steve, or she'll make such a fuss," Sabrina pleaded.

"OK. When I finish with Mr. Kennedy. But tell her I only have a few minutes. By the way, did you check under the mink?"

Sabrina giggled. "She's not wearing it today; it's too warm. Just a simple little frock, so it's A-OK."

I went back to Kato. He had spent the night in the clinic after having eaten the better part of his owner's fresh-caught ten-pound cod. "As long as he's here, why don't I give him his booster shot? He's due for it next week anyway. Save you the trip."

Mr. Kennedy peered at me over his steel-rimmed bifocals. He was a tall, skinny man of about sixty-five, with a ruddy, weathered face and a long, well-lined neck that stuck up from the buttoned collar of his tieless white shirt. "Why not? He's had everything else here. I have to bust the bank every time I bring him in. This damned cat costs more than bringing up three kids."

"Aw come on, Mr. Kennedy," I cajoled. "You know he's worth it. He's a real beauty." With difficulty, I pulled the twenty-two pound cat down from around my neck and planted him firmly on the exam table. He was an enormous black and white Maine Coon, a rare breed I had never seen before I met Kato. The cat's bushy black tail flicked my face and his oval golden eyes looked up at me inscrutably. He purred like a well-oiled machine and rubbed up against my lab coat.

"He is kind of special, I guess." Mr. Kennedy's craggy face cracked in a smile. "Ya know he sleeps in the bed with us now. My wife's nuts about him. If I was a little younger, I'd be jealous of the damned cat."

I administered the shot in the ruff of the cat's neck. Kato mewed softly and Mr. Kennedy winced.

"There you go Kato old boy, no fish bones, no long claws, no mysterious diseases. All finished until the next time." I rubbed his neck briskly, then handed him to Mr. Kennedy, who ever so gently placed him in a large cat carrier and carefully closed and locked the see-through lid.

"Don't know that I should be thanking you, since I'm the one's leaving my bankbook here. Seems you should be thanking me."

"Thank you, Mr. Kennedy," I said dutifully. "Sabrina has your bill out front."

He grumped at me by way of good-bye, hoisted the carrier so

that Kato's large head bobbed behind the clear plastic, making him look like a pasha being carried in an enclosed litter, and was out the door.

When he had gone, I sprayed the exam table with antiseptic and straightened the row of disposable syringes on the white Formica counter. As treatment rooms go, this one was extremely pleasant. A shaft of sun shone through the Plexiglas skylight directly onto the exam table below, heightening the cheeriness of the bright yellow walls. White Formica medicine cabinets and a built-in sink lined one side of the room and on the other was a low, soldier-blue cushioned bench for clients. The walls were bare except for two diplomas framed in Plexiglas, mine from Michigan State School of Veterinary Medicine and George Carney's from the University of Pennsylvania School of Veterinary Medicine. A swinging door at the far end of the room led to the neat, white-tiled surgery next door and beyond that, a duplicate treatment room.

I sat down on the client bench for a moment to gather my strength for Mrs. Wyman. I would need it. I decided to ask Sabrina to stay in the room with us when I saw her. It would be safer that way. To be honest, Mrs. Wyman scared the hell out of me. It was hard to tell how old she was. She'd had her face lifted, I was certain of that, because it had that masklike, plumped-up look, and she was always heavily made up. But I judged her to be somewhere in her late fifties.

According to Sabrina, Mr. Wyman had made a fortune by inventing a sealing process for frozen foods. He stashed his wife in a big mansion outside of Lexington, with a full complement of servants, and went his own way, making more money, I supposed, or maybe just trying to put as much distance as possible between him and Mrs. Wyman. As far as George Carney was concerned, she was a terrific client. She had two animals, the malamute dog and a Himalayan cat, and she was in the clinic with one or the other of them at least once a week. She never made an appointment; it was always an emergency visit. The dog couldn't move its leg, or the cat had swallowed its toy. But when I examined the animal, I never could find anything wrong.

Since I was the one she insisted handle the case, I was convinced she made up the symptoms as an excuse to see me. Before I came to work here, I never would have thought that. Women didn't pursue me. In fact, with the girls I dated it was just the opposite. But after my first week at George Carney's clinic, it seemed that a network of Indian drums was brought into play, and we were suddenly besieged by new women clients, all of whom wanted me to treat their animals. Combining diplomacy with humor, I could handle most of them, but Mrs. Wyman was another story.

What was a supposition became a certainty the day Mrs. Wyman sailed into the clinic wrapped in mink and a cloud of heavy perfume, carrying Tulip, the cat. Tulip, she announced, was choking and had to be seen immediately, by me, of course. George, who envisioned dollar bills floating in front of his eyes whenever he saw her, took over the case I was handling, and I was left with Mrs. Wyman and Tulip.

I took the cat from her arms and placed her on the exam table. Tulip was strikingly beautiful. A nearly perfect Himalayan, her coat was a thick, silky, bluish white, with blue points on her ears, nose and luxuriously bushy tail. Her eyes were deep blue, the color of the cushion on the clients' bench. They closed as she purred contentedly. There was no sign of choking or coughing. To be absolutely sure, I opened her mouth and peered down her throat with a flashlight. There was no obstruction; everything was perfectly normal.

When I began the examination, Mrs. Wyman was on the other side of the table. By the time I finished looking in the cat's throat, she was at my side. Her perfume was overpowering. I moved farther down the table, sliding Tulip along with me.

"Mrs. Wyman, there's nothing wrong with Tulip that I can see," I sputtered nervously, trying to stay away from her. The table was only six feet long. I had reached the end and I moved around to the other side. She followed, her hand now on my arm.

"How can that be? I just don't understand it. Dear Dr. Kritsick," she said in a low voice. Her hand moved up my arm to my neck and then my ear lobe. "She was coughing and choking so

badly, poor thing, I thought sure she'd die." Mrs. Wyman moved
closer. "You have wonderful hair, dear, dear, Dr. Kritsick. Did
anyone ever tell you what wonderful, heavy, dark hair you have?
Men with heavy, dark hair are always so— so—potent!"

Before I could pull away again, her hand had traveled up my
neck and into my hair. I left Tulip on the table and stood by the
sink. I tried to think about George's dollar signs and not say anything to hurt her feelings.

"I think if you took Tulip home now, she'd be just fine." I
started to reach for the cat, who was still purring loudly with her
eyes closed, but Mrs. Wyman placed herself between me and the
table.

"You're such an attractive young man, dear Dr. Kritsick, and I
could do such wonderful things for you—to you."

She backed me up against the sink so that my head was pushing into the cabinet above. Suddenly, she was all over me. Her
hands were underneath my lab coat, working feverishly down my
chest to my waist and then to my legs. I couldn't scream for help.
After all, I was bigger than she was. I pushed her away as gently
as I could and made for the other side of the room. If I could just
get to the door. But she was faster and she got there before me,
leaning against it, barring my exit.

"Don't run away from me, you sweet boy. I can make you so,
so happy. Listen how my heart beats for you." In a thrice, she
had the listening ends of my stethoscope in my ears and the other
end against her chest. I heard one thump before I yanked the ear
pieces out of my ears and retreated back to the table. I picked up
Tulip and was about to push Mrs. Wyman aside and flee out the
door, when she tugged at the belt on her mink coat. It opened
and the folds of the coat fell away, revealing all of George Carney's most lucrative client. She was stark naked underneath. She
posed for a moment, batting her heavily mascaraed eyes at me. I
was so flustered I didn't quite know what to do. I felt my face
flush, not because I'm a prude, but because I was embarrassed
and sorry for her all at once.

I didn't say anything. I put the cat down and gently belted the
coat around Mrs. Wyman, put my arm around her, scooped up

Tulip again and escorted them both to the client's outer door. Her car and chauffeur were waiting. When I put the cat in her arms, she swept straight to the car without speaking and without looking back. She got in and it drove away.

Sabrina had watched the procession from her desk with great interest and, when I told her what had happened, she, of course, understood even better than I how sad Mrs. Wyman was. But we were only human, and soon we were both dissolved in gales of laughter, as I described being chased around the treatment room. We laughed so hard we couldn't speak, and tears were rolling down our faces. When George came out to ask what had happened, we could only point and make incomprehensible signs. It was fully five minutes before we were actually able to tell him about the unfortunate demise of his hoped-for future wealth.

It had been over two months since we'd heard from Mrs. Wyman. Now she was back again, and I dreaded the encounter. Best to have it over with as quickly as possible so I could get to lunch. I buzzed Sabrina on the intercom. "Send Mrs. Wyman in, and why don't you come along with her?" I asked plaintively.

"Don't you think that's a little obvious, Steve?" Sabrina whispered. "You're a big boy, you can handle it." She clicked off before I could say anything else.

I was standing at the exam table when Mrs. Wyman came into the room. Harold, her malamute, preceded her on a long lead. I was surprised to see he was actually limping. Mrs. Wyman wore a simple but expensive silk shirt dress in a deep hunter green, with a sort of cinnamon-colored stripe on the collar and sleeve cuffs. Her purse and shoes matched the stripe exactly. Her makeup was understated. Without all the mascara, I could see her eyes for the first time. They were a deep green, almost the same color as her dress. Her blond hair was cut short and curled softly so that it framed her face. Whether that was its natural color or not, I didn't know. Her manner was quiet and calm. There was no hint of the frantic sexuality she had projected before. I realized she was a very attractive woman. I tried to behave as professionally as possible. I would make no reference to our last meeting and I hoped that she wouldn't either.

She put her purse down on the bench and knelt next to her dog. "He's got something the matter with his paw, doctor. I've looked, but I can't see anything, and he's been limping for three days."

I knelt in front of Harold, stroked his head and patted his flank. Even though I had seen him several times before, with dogs it's always a good idea to talk to them before you treat them. He was a big dog, weighing close to ninety pounds, with the fierce masklike markings of the malamute and cold blue eyes that harked back to his wolf ancestors. But in fact, they belied his gentle disposition. Harold was a pussycat.

"Hey boy, that's a good fella. Let's see that gimpy paw. I'm not gonna hurt you. You know that, don't you?" I lifted his right front paw and flexed it. There was no broken bone. "Let's get him up on the table under the light." Mrs. Wyman made a move to help. "No, no, I can manage," I told her. I held the dog under his chest and hind paws and hoisted him onto the table, not without some effort.

"OK, big fella, let's see what the problem is. Sit, Harold," I commanded gently. Harold obeyed immediately, and I lifted his paw to the light so that I could see between the pads. "Aha! There's the little bugger." It was a small needle from some kind of burr. Difficult to see without very good light. I got a hemostat from the counter, inserted the points between the pads and quickly pulled the needle out. Harold whimpered, but not too loudly. I held the almost infinitesimal needle up for Mrs. Wyman to see. "There it is. That's what was doing the damage. You'll be fine now, Harold. I guarantee it."

"Just like Androcles and the lion. Now he'll be your friend forever," Mrs. Wyman said, petting her dog fondly.

"I certainly hope so." I washed the paw with antiseptic, gave Harold a shot of an antibiotic to prevent any infection and lifted him down off the table. Glad to be finished with it, the dog wagged his tail appreciatively.

"He's certainly grateful, doctor, and I am too. Thank you." She extended her hand and I took it. This was not the same woman who had been in here two months ago, not physically and certainly not mentally. What had happened to her in the interim I didn't know, but the new Mrs. Wyman was a distinct improvement. I wondered if she even knew there *was* an old Mrs. Wyman. Perhaps she had blocked it out, like Joanne Woodward in *The Three Faces of Eve*. It had to be something like that. People can't change that radically in just two months, or can they?

When she had gone, I hurriedly washed my hands and changed my lab coat for a sports jacket. It was almost 12:30. I was going to be late for lunch. I raced out the treatment-room door and ran smack into Sabrina.

"You weren't going to leave without telling me what happened, were you?" Her eyebrow was raised accusingly.

"No, but I'm late for lunch. I'll tell you when I get back."

"She didn't attack you, did she." It was more a statement than a question.

"No, she didn't. How did you know?"

"I just knew. She seemed different this time—like another person."

"She was. We'll talk about it later. I think it's kind of interesting." I was halfway out the front door.

"Have a good lunch," she called after me.

I got into my car to drive the five miles to The Yankee Peddlar Inn, an old grist mill converted to a restaurant, on the other side of Lexington. It was a pretty spot, full of tourist-book charm, but few tourists knew about it. It had an open dining terrace overlooking a stream, and today would be warm enough to eat outside. I hoped that if David got there first, he would be bright enough to get a terrace table. Since David had joined a law practice in Concord, we didn't get to lunch together that often. But when we did, The Yankee Peddlar was the place we liked best, because they had terrific homemade desserts. I could almost taste the cherry cobbler.

I rolled down the windows of the car and breathed in the balmy spring air. It was a glorious day, almost too warm for my jacket. The trees were just about in full leaf; another few weeks and it would be summer. Nothing excited me more than the thought of summer and our weekends at the Cape. I accelerated the car, and it groaned with the extra exertion. It was a six-year-old Plymouth and it bore the scars of the wear and tear I had given it. I'm very hard on a car, and this one rattled and sighed with every turn of the wheel. If I could talk George Carney into a raise, perhaps I'd be able to trade it in on a new one in the fall.

I pulled into the restaurant parking lot and found a place right next to the door. David was already there. I spotted his prized 1966 red Mustang convertible parked down the line. He had restored it completely, and it was probably worth a fortune now. I should learn to take better care of my cars. Perhaps I would do better with the next one.

I was ten minutes late. David was usually early, so that when I arrived anywhere on time, he was already tapping his toe. I raced through the inn's barn-siding paneled dining room. In winter, it was crowded with people, all vying for tables near, or within sight of, the huge stone fireplace that reached across the entire front wall. Today, it was empty except for waiters running back and forth from the kitchen. Shafts of sunlight poured into the room through the open French doors that led to the large stone terrace. There, the twenty-odd tables were occupied by diners, seated under big, bright, blue-and-white umbrellas. The clatter of silver and the lively hum of voices mingled with the rushing sound of the mill stream and the waterfall nearby.

I saw David at a corner table for two, on the far side of the terrace next to the railing. He was all dressed up in his three-piece lawyer suit, looking very successful, if a little somber. The sunlight was just hitting his table as I came in, and he reached into his breast pocket and put on a pair of dark glasses. Of medium height, he was slender, but well muscled. Even sitting down, he had the look of a trained athlete, which he was. David had been a track star at college and next year he was planning to run in the Boston Marathon.

He was toying with the little plastic straw from his drink, trying to fit one end into the other. When I slipped into the seat opposite him, he looked up briefly and then went back to the straw, without bothering to greet me.

"Sorry I'm late. Had a last-minute patient. You been waiting long?"

"A few minutes," he said, not looking up.

I signaled the waiter and ordered a beer. "Do you want another drink?" I asked, noticing his was almost finished.

"Uh-uh," he shook his head.

I couldn't see his eyes behind the dark glasses, but I knew something was wrong. "Hey, what's the matter? Did you lose a case or something? Don't I even rate a hello? I'm really sorry about being late, I just couldn't help it."

He just sat there, fiddling with the little plastic straw from his drink. The waiter brought my beer and asked if we wanted to order lunch. I told him we'd wait a few minutes and turned to David again. "Jesus, David, it's the most beautiful day of the year. Finally, we're gonna do what we've talked about for years. Finally, we're gonna have a summer house of our very own so we won't have to scrounge every damned weekend from other people, and you're sitting there moping. Now what the hell's the matter with you? What's wrong? Tell me."

His mouth quivered as he tried to hold back the tears. "I'm gonna die, Steve."

I felt a stab of fear, but I pushed it away. "I'm gonna die too. We're all gonna die someday, so what else is new?" Maybe he was having an attack of spring melancholia. David didn't do things like that, but there was always a first time. I'd just have to josh him out of it. "Come on, it's too pretty out to talk about dying. I get flashes of it sometimes too. Everybody does. But if you thought about it all the time, you'd go nuts. Why don't we order lunch and talk about the Cape and . . ."

He reached across the table and grabbed my hand. "Listen to me, Steve. Please, listen!" He took his dark glasses off. The color was drained from his face. His eyes were bloodshot and brimming with tears. "I'm not talking about someday. I'm not talking about flashes. I'm talking about now—soon! I went to the doctor this morning."

"What doctor?" I was incredulous. How could this be happening?

"Hamilton at Mass. General."

"In Boston? Why didn't you go to Weiner?"

"I did. He sent me to Hamilton."

"Why?"

"He's a specialist. For God's sake, Steve, will you let me finish!"

I realized I was interrupting out of nervousness. "I'm sorry, tell me the whole story from the beginning."

David took a deep breath. "Remember I had those chest pains? The ones we thought came from lifting the weights?"

I nodded, recalling my initial off-the-top-of-the-head home diagnosis.

"Well, they got worse."

"Why didn't you say anything? I talk to you almost every day."

"What could you do? Besides, I thought you were right and they'd go away if I stopped lifting the weights. But they didn't. Finally, they got so bad I went to see Weiner yesterday. He thumped and listened and X-rayed and told me I should see Hamilton immediately. I asked him what he thought was wrong, but you know how these damned doctors are, they never like to commit themselves. He said he wasn't sure, but there might be a little obstruction in my chest and he wanted Hamilton to have a look—he's a chest specialist. He said he'd call him himself and make the appointment for me because he wanted me seen as soon as possible. I was a little scared, but I figured, what the hell, it couldn't be very much. Anyway, I went in and saw Hamilton at nine this morning. He took more X rays." He stopped for breath. He was holding my hand so tightly it hurt. "Oh Jesus, I'm so frightened, Steve!"

I put my other hand on his arm, trying to calm him. I knew instinctively what he was going to tell me and I didn't want to hear. "What did he say, David? Tell me!"

He took another deep breath, and a tear escaped from his eye and trickled down his cheek. He brushed it away quickly.

"He said there are two masses in my chest that could be malignant. He wanted to admit me to the hospital right then and there, to make tests and see if there are any more anyplace else. I said I needed to go home first. I promised to be back at four this afternoon." He took his hand away and slumped back in the chair. "I don't want to die. It's not fair. I'm not even twenty-five."

The saliva in my mouth suddenly tasted funny and metallic, like I was going to throw up. My fingers and toes tingled, as if all the blood had left my body. If I had been standing, I might have fallen down. The sounds around me, of people laughing, glasses and silver clinking, the roar of the waterfall, were surrealistic and far away.

I had thought about death before, but in flashes, like I told David. It was distant and poetic. It happened to other people, friends of my parents, Grandpa Ernest, when I was five. A girl in high school slipped through the ice and drowned. When I was nineteen and working in Mt. Auburn Hospital, a boy my own age died of cancer. But not me, not someone I was really close to. I put animals to sleep all the time. That was an odd euphemism—putting an animal to sleep. I was killing it. It died. But that was different, or was it? Death is death. David would die, I would die.

All at once, I felt embarrassed. I was intruding on a secret place. David's new secret place, not yet mine. We had always shared everything. How could we now share this? Did I want to? If he was my friend, I had to. But how? Maybe it wasn't true. Doctors have been wrong before, just like vets can be wrong. The thought comforted me enough that I could speak again.

"Listen, Hamilton isn't God. He could be wrong, you know. And you're just going in for tests, you'll be out in a couple of days."

"I saw the X rays, Steve. I saw the tumors," David said quietly. "They're pretty big."

"OK, so what's the worst? They'll operate, get those buggers out and you'll recuperate for the rest of the summer down at the Cape. Not so awful." I was lying. If there were two tumors and they were large, chances were they were malignant, and if they had metastasized—but I couldn't think about that.

"Have you told your folks?"

"No, I thought I'd wait till after lunch. I have to go home and get a bathrobe, pajamas and stuff. I thought I'd tell my mother then. You know how she is, she'll cry and then run to church. I didn't want to worry her until I knew what it was. But since I have to go to the hospital, I guess I better tell her. Maybe I should call my dad first. Maybe he ought to be there when I tell her. What do you think?"

"I think that's a good idea. Do you want me to call him for you?"

He thought for a moment. "No, I'd better do it myself. Dad's pretty good about this kind of thing."

David's father was a fireman. When we were little, he took us for rides on the hook-and-ladder engine, which made us special and privileged among our friends. I liked Mr. Hennessey. He was a big, gruff Irishman and, since David and I were always at each other's houses, he treated me like another son. I hoped David was right. I hoped Mr. Hennessey could handle it. After all, he was used to emergencies. Except they were always other people's. It was David's mother I was really worried about. She was a small, fragile woman whose entire life was wrapped up in her son. She had taught school until David finished law school, so that there would be enough money for his tuition. When he graduated, she was so proud, you would've thought she had gone through every class with him. I hated to think how she would react to his news. I could only hope she wouldn't make it harder for him than it already was. Although worrying about her might help him take his mind off himself.

"Steve, would you mind if we didn't eat any lunch? I don't much feel like it."

"I don't either. Why don't you go call your dad from here while I take care of the check."

When David left I looked at the stream below. A pair of ducks followed by four fuzzy ducklings scooted by, the mother duck honking to lead the way. The trees were burgeoning with bright green new leaves. Everything was so fresh and alive, there was no room for death on such a day. It came to me that perhaps I was having a terrible nightmare and, somehow, I had to wake myself up. I slammed my hand against the rail as hard as I could. The pain was so intense, I doubled over, clutching my hand between my legs to stop it.

"What did you do? Did you hurt yourself?" a familiar voice said. I looked up to see that David had returned. It wasn't a dream.

"No, it's nothing. I just whanged my hand by mistake. Did you get your dad?"

"Yeah, he's gonna meet me at home now."

"Did you tell him the whole story?"

"Sort of. He was pretty upset, but I think he'll be OK. It's Mom I don't want to tell. Maybe I shouldn't until we're really sure. What do you think?" David seemed much calmer now that he had his parents to be concerned about.

"I don't know," I answered, after a moment.

We walked through the dining room out to the parking lot. I thought about how it would be if I had to tell my own mother. Not terrific, that's for sure. But my mother's a realist. She'd want to know. I think she'd feel much worse if I hid something like this from her. Then again, maybe we were underestimating Mrs. Hennessey; maybe she'd want to know too.

"I guess you ought to tell your mom—at least what you know so far. She's gonna find out anyway and she might be hurt if she felt you didn't think she was strong enough to handle it."

"Yeah, maybe," David mumbled.

We had reached the red Mustang. It was so shiny, you could use it to shave by. And why not? David never stopped polishing his aging prize. He took off his jacket, hung it neatly on the hook. He rolled down the window, got into the car and closed the door.

I bent down and leaned on the open window. "Will you be all right? Do you want me to come home with you?" I made the offer hoping he'd refuse. I didn't want to be there when he told his mother.

"Nah, I'll be OK. Don't worry, I'm not an invalid yet."

"I know you're not. That's not what I meant," I started to explain and then thought better of it. "OK, drive carefully and I'll see you at the hospital. I'll be there right after work."

"You don't have to do that, you really don't. I'll be fine, honest!"

"I know you will. I just want to be there. Is that OK with you?"' There was a tinge of impatience in my voice, almost as if I were talking to a child. David picked up on it.

"Of course it is. You know I want you there. It's just that I know how tired you are after work and I didn't want you to have to schlepp all the way into Boston."

"It's no problem," I assured him.

"Thanks." He smiled. His hair had fallen in his eyes, making him look more seventeen than twenty-five, though I noticed the dark circles under his eyes.

He started the car and gunned the engine, listening with satisfaction to its strong purring sound. Then he looked up at me again. "Steve, one more thing—" He took a deep breath. "Do you really think they can get those things out of my chest?"

"Of course they can," I answered immediately. "I do it all the time on my dogs and cats, and they're running around to tell about it. It's a cinch!" Once more, I lied.

He nodded. Whether he accepted my answer or not, I didn't know. Without saying anything further he backed the car out of its parking place and drove out of the lot. I was to see him in that shiny red Mustang only once more.

That day was better than ten months ago. David had been dead since January, and still the awful feeling wouldn't go away. A strong, biting wind had come up on the bridge, and I was suddenly very cold. When I looked at my watch, I realized I had been staring at the water for over half an hour. If I was to be on time for my nine o'clock patient, I'd have to quicken my pace back to the clinic. I jogged in place for a few minutes, trying to get my blood going again, and started back down the road.

I warmed up as I ran, trying to think about anything but David, but I couldn't get him out of my mind.

After the tests, which involved biopsy surgery of the chest tumors, it was discovered that his cancer had begun in the lymph glands. The killer cells had metastasized, not only to his chest, but throughout his body. The prognosis from the beginning was grim. And, unfortunately, he was young and strong, so it took him longer to die.

Since further surgery would accomplish nothing, a program of chemotherapy was instituted that was probably just as futile. However, it gave us all a slender thread of hope to cling to, everyone that is, but David. He knew at the start, his life, brief as it was, was over. He had accepted death and, when the pain became unbearable, welcomed it.

Mrs. Hennessey, on the other hand, was certain her son would be miraculously cured, and when she wasn't at the hospital she spent all of her time in St. Francis's Church, praying for his recovery. Her faith carried her through the ordeal, but it couldn't save her son. Mr. Hennessey, though he didn't share his wife's unshaken faith, was able to sustain himself simply by denying the fact that his son would die. He was always talking about what they would do, where they would go and how it would be when David got out of the hospital.

And I, with all my medical knowledge, even I hoped for a miracle. As I watched his body deteriorate, as I saw his blond hair fall out with the chemotherapy, as I saw the searing pain each time he breathed, I too hoped for a miraculous remission. That wasn't so farfetched. Things like that had happened before. Medically inexplicable, it just happens. Suddenly, a dying person is better. Why not David?

Then in early August, it did happen. For no apparent reason, his breathing eased and the pain lessened. I had been coming to the hospital almost every day since he was admitted and knew his doctors well. Why not, I suggested, let me take him out of the hospital just for the weekend. I'd drive him down to the Cape and bring him back early Sunday evening. If anything went wrong, I'd have him back sooner. They agreed.

When I told David my idea, his eyes lit up, but then a look of nervous apprehension flickered over his thin, hollow face. He was sitting up in bed, eating his dinner. It was the first time in weeks he'd had any appetite.

"I don't know, Steve. I don't want anyone to see me like this.

Kenny and Joe probably will have people there, and I don't want to see anyone, not even them." He had finished his lamb chop and was now eating his Jell-O with relish.

I looked at him. Except for small fuzzy patches, almost all his hair had fallen out. He was so thin, I could encircle his upper arm with my hand. His eyes, though clear and very blue that day, were sunken in his head.

I thought quickly. "Do you think I'm a dummy? Did you think I wouldn't know that? Kenny and Joe are going to a wedding this weekend. The house will be empty; it's all ours," I lied again. I was getting very good at it, almost glib. I would call Kenny and Joe and ask them—no, tell them—to give us the house for the weekend. I knew they couldn't refuse, and as it turned out, they didn't.

On that Saturday morning, I pulled up in front of Mass. General in David's red Mustang. Not only was my car in no shape to make the trip to the Cape, but I knew how pleased he would be to ride in the Mustang again. I had carefully polished and waxed every inch of it so that it gleamed from front bumper to taillight, something I had never done for my own poor, abused heap.

David was waiting at the entrance in a wheelchair, his nurse at his side. This was the first time I had seen him in street clothes in over three months. They badly accentuated his emaciated frame. His arms hung out of his short-sleeved Hawaiian sport shirt like pipe cleaners, and even with him sitting down, I could see that his khaki trousers were at least three sizes too big. On his head, he had perched an inverted white sailor cap at a rakish angle so that it hid the remaining tufts of hair on his almost bald scalp. His nurse handed me a plastic bag filled with his medication, including liquid demerol for pain, and explained how and when each thing should be administered. She helped me get David into the front seat, and we collapsed the wheelchair and put it in the trunk. With my usual optimism, I hoped we wouldn't need it.

The two-hour drive down to the Cape was uneventful. David dozed most of the way, awakening every half hour to ask, like a child, if we were there yet, then nodding off again. I drove carefully and defensively, taking pains to avoid short stops, or cars that seemed to have erratic drivers. I wanted David to have this weekend without any mishaps.

He was still sleeping when I turned off Route 6 onto the smaller Route 28, which led to Chatham. That's where the shack was. It belonged to Joe's aunt, and since she was to be in California for the summer, she'd agreed to let us all rent it for a very small fee. When she heard what had happened to David, she let Joe and Kenny have it for even less. Otherwise, there was no way any of us could have afforded a house right on the beach. In the last ten years, real estate in that area had become frightfully expensive. It cost a small fortune to rent even the smallest shack, especially if it was on the water.

I turned down the long, winding dirt road that led to the shack. It was filled with ruts and bumps that I couldn't avoid. David woke up when I hit a particularly nasty one.

"That's pretty good timing, pal; we're here." I turned the car into the rough gravel driveway at the rear of the shack. "How do you feel? You don't look any worse than when we started."

"That's not saying much." David grinned.

"Sit here for a minute and let me get things organized," I told him, pushing the driver's seat forward to get my duffle and his small overnight bag out of the backseat. I slung them up on the porch and opened the trunk to get the wheelchair and the bag of medicine. I unfolded the chair and pushed it around to David's side of the car.

"I think it'll be easier if I walk. You'll never be able to hoist that damned thing up the steps," he said.

"OK, if you think you can. But first let me open the house so we can go right in."

I took the ignition key from the car—I had attached the house key to it so I wouldn't lose or misplace it, as I've been known to do—and bounded up the steps of the back porch. The house was an old saltbox that had been added on to over the years. The back porch was a recent addition that Joe, David and I had helped to build three summers ago. It was more a small deck than a porch, but Joe's aunt liked to think of it as a porch, and we went along with her.

I put the key in the rusty lock and jiggled it a few times until it finally creaked and turned the tumbler. When I opened the door, I was engulfed in that musty, slightly mildew smell that goes with all summer cottages by the sea. Joe and Kenny had left the kitchen neat as a pin. There was a note on the refrigerator telling me there was enough food in the freezer to last the weekend, so I wouldn't have to leave David to shop. They had thought of everything.

I walked through the kitchen to the large living room. At one end, sliding glass doors opened onto a deck that overlooked the beach and, farther down, the sea. At the other end of the room was a big brick fireplace. Wood was stacked on either side of the mantel as well as in a kind of shelf cut into the wall adjoining it. The room was simply but comfortably furnished, with a white-cushioned wicker couch and two matching wicker club chairs. A hooked rug covered the center of the wide-planked floor, and in front of the couch was a coffee table made from an old sea chest. The walls were painted white and adorned with the treasures of countless summers. A piece of driftwood over the couch, a pair of duck decoys on the mantel, a brass ship's bell near the window and a framed water color done by someone who had evidently lived in the house. Shells of every known bivalve and mollusk in the area littered the room's tables and shelves, serving as ashtrays and catchalls.

Off to each side of the living room were the bedrooms, three in all. The master bedroom, to the right, had twin beds and an adjoining bath. It too had sliding glass doors opening onto the deck. I thought that would be the best room for David. I put his small bag on one bed and turned down the covers on the other. I would take one of the smaller rooms on the other side of the house, unless he didn't want to be by himself.

I opened the doors in the bedroom and then in the living room, to let the fresh sea air blow through the house, and went back outside to fetch David. He was waiting patiently for me.

"It's terrific," I told him. "Joe and Kenny are great housekeepers. They even left us food in the fridge for the weekend. Now, let's get you inside. Are you sure you want to walk?"

"I'd like to give it a try," he said. He'd been sitting in the car, with the door open and his legs hanging outside.

"OK, let me help you up." I got my shoulder under his arm and lifted him to his feet. He shuffled a few feet and then collapsed against me.

"Guess I'm not as sturdy as I thought."

"Of course you are. You're just not used to walking. I'll carry you in, and then we'll take it a little at a time. Put your arms around my neck." I grabbed him under the legs and carried him up the steps. He weighed no more than a child. I went straight into the bedroom and laid him on the bed.

"There you go, service with a smile. The view is great and the price is right. What more could you ask?"

"Maybe another summer," he said quietly.

I pretended not to hear. "Hey, listen, the best thing in the world for you is some sun and fresh air. Sun, that's what you need. Sun fixes everything." I grabbed a pillow from the bed and put it on the chaise on the deck outside the bedroom door. David was struggling into his shorts. I could see it took almost all of his energy to stand up and pull them over his hips.

"It'll be better if I carry you." I lifted him easily and walked the few steps to the deck, placing him gently on the chaise.

"You're getting very good at this, nurse."

"Listen Hennessey, I'm not gonna make a career of it, so don't get any fancy ideas." I laughed, and for the first time, he laughed too.

The air was hot and dry, but the breeze from the sea made it feel soft and comforting on the skin. At another time, I would have thought how good it was to be alive. In fact, I did think that. How good it was to be alive and healthy. Then I looked at David and felt terribly guilty. I was constantly aware of him reading my mind. Mostly, it was my imagination. But every once in a while, he'd say something that made me know I was right. I suppose it had to do with my acceptance, finally, that he was going to die and I was going to live. Like the survivors of concentration camps who suffered so intensely because others were sent to the ovens and they weren't. It's an odd feeling, a combination of relief: thank God it's not me, and guilt: oh God, why him and not me?

"Do you want a Coke or something to eat before I park myself?" It was just noon; I figured we'd have lunch in an hour or so.

"No, I'm fine. Sit down for a while. I've been thinking about something a lot and I want to talk with you." He looked serious.

I plopped down on the chair, my face turned toward the sun. It felt hot and good. "Shoot!" I said, with my eyes closed.

"Do you remember that summer you worked at Mt. Auburn Hospital, before you went to vet school? Remember you thought you might change your mind and go to med school after all?"

"Yeah, so?"

"Well, you could still do it. You're only twenty-five, it's not too late."

I did remember. I was nineteen and had finagled a job as an operating-room scrub technician at Mt. Auburn the summer after my freshman year at Michigan State. It was exciting work, and I was good at it. Certainly the life-and-death drama of the operating room turned my head a bit, and when Dr. Halloway, the Chief of Surgery, suggested that he would recommend me to Harvard Med School, of course I was flattered and considered it for a while. But just for a while. Then Peter Schiller was brought into the O.R. with testicular cancer. He was nineteen that summer too. They operated on him, and before I left for school in September, he was dead. I watched him die, just as I was watching David, and there was nothing I or anyone else could do to help him. It was a searing experience. All the more so because I was so young and identified with him in the same way I did now with David, even though I didn't know Peter well.

My grades were good, and I probably would have been accepted in med school, but I knew then I didn't want a career in human medicine. The failure rate was too high.

"I don't think so, David. I love what I'm doing, you know that."

"Yeah, but if you became a doctor, maybe you could help people like me."

"You've got the best in the business working for you. If I were a doctor, I doubt I could do any better." I looked over at him, avoiding his real point. He was peering at me from under that silly sailor hat, which had slid over his eyes.

"I don't know. I guess I just would like to think you were doing something really worthwhile with your life, that's all."

"But what I do *is* worthwhile. Animals are a part of life. I love them, always have loved them, and I feel I contribute a lot by helping them."

"Don't you love people?"

"Of course I do, David."

What I wanted to say was, if I were a doctor and knew there was nothing I could do—that a case was hopeless—the frustration would have been unbearable.

"Why don't you at least think about it," he persisted.

"OK, I'll think about it. In the meantime, how about some lunch?"

"I'm not really hungry now. You have something."

"I'm gonna fix us my famous tuna-salad sandwiches. When you see them, you won't be able to resist."

I left him on the deck and went into the kitchen, as much to be by myself for a minute as to make the sandwiches. When I first thought about taking David away for the weekend, I knew it would be difficult, but I had thought only about the physical difficulties. The fact that it would be such an emotional wrench never occurred to me.

I puttered about, opening and closing cabinets, to find cans of tuna and the Miracle Whip. There were some beautiful tomatoes in a bowl on the kitchen table. I sliced one, added it to the sandwiches, poured a beer for myself and a Coke for David, and put it all on a tray and carried it out to the deck.

I had been gone only ten minutes. If he called me, I hadn't heard him. He had tried to get up from the chaise and had fallen. His sailor cap had come off and lay next to his almost hairless head.

"Oh Christ, Steve, help me! It's hurting so much."

He was having difficulty breathing. Why hadn't I thought to ask for an oxygen unit? I picked him up and carried him back into the bedroom. He was bathed in perspiration, his eyes clouded with pain. His breath came in short rasping bursts.

"Oh God, God!" he screamed. "It's like knives in there. Please give me something quick. Please, Steve. Something's inside my chest chewing on me."

I ran to the plastic bag with the medication and pulled out the bottle of liquid demerol and a syringe. I filled it with 2 cc's and injected it intramuscularly in his upper arm.

"OK, Davey. It'll stop in a minute. Try and take a deep breath."

The tears streamed down his face. "I can't, Steve, it hurts too much."

"Count to ten. Just count to ten and it'll stop. I promise."

Liquid demerol worked quickly. It wouldn't kill the pain completely, but David would just float above it. At least it would be bearable. He was obediently counting, saying each number through clenched teeth, and by the time he reached eight, his face was no longer contorted, his frail body had relaxed. What worried me was his breathing. It was still harsh and rasping.

I had made a terrible mistake. The trip was too much for him. The remission, such as it was, hadn't lasted long enough to give him this final weekend. It would be foolish to stay here any longer. If his condition became really complicated, I couldn't handle it. The only choice was to get him back to Mass. General as quickly as possible.

He had fallen into an uneasy drugged sleep, moaning with pain, yet not conscious of it. The effects of the demerol in his bloodstream would last no more than three hours, barely enough time for the ride back.

I packed up our gear and stowed it in the trunk of the Mustang, along with the wheelchair. All that remained was to call the hospital and tell them David was coming back. When I had done that, I went to the bedroom. David was sleeping soundly. I lifted him as gently as I could, carried him out to the car and laid him in the backseat. Under his head I placed a pillow I had taken from the house, and I covered him with a knitted afghan.

The rutted dirt road seemed even rougher and bumpier than

when we drove in. I tried to navigate it so that David wouldn't feel the inevitable bouncing. As sleek a car as it was, the Mustang was never noted for the comfort of its backseat. Maybe I should've called for an ambulance. Too late for that now. We were almost at Route 6, the Cape highway. David moaned. I looked over my shoulder, he was restless and trying to turn in the seat. Please don't fall off, Davey, I beg of you, please!

When I turned onto Route 6, it was jammed with traffic. What else did I expect on a beautiful Saturday in August. I wove in and out of traffic lanes, trying to make time. I was being the kind of driver I hated, but there was nothing for it. I had to hurry. If a cop stopped me, I'd just tell him David was in the backseat dying. Then maybe I'd have a motorcycle escort. The drama of that thought carried me clear to Route 3, past Plymouth and Pembroke.

We had been traveling for about two and a half hours and had almost reached Quincy, on the outskirts of Boston, when David came to. I had the accelerator practically down to the floor. We were doing at least eighty-five when I heard him scream. It so unnerved me, I damned near went off the road.

"Hang in there, Davey. Just another few minutes and we'll be back at the hospital. Just hang in there."

"I can't, Steve. It hurts too much."

"Yes, you can," I said over my shoulder. "Just five more minutes and it'll be all over. Five minutes and you'll be back in your bed and they'll give you whatever you want. I promise."

I couldn't stop now; it was only a matter of minutes. But every time he screamed, my heart stopped. How long was this pain to continue? How long would they let him linger on? How many shots of demerol and then, when that no longer worked, how many shots of morphine? At least the animals I treated didn't have to suffer. There were no lingering deaths. I could do for dogs and cats what no doctor could do for David. I could end suffering for my patients. I could put them to sleep. If only I could do that for my best friend.

I pulled into the emergency entrance of Mass. General, ran out of the car and got the emergency team with a rolling stretcher.

They lifted David out, placed him on the stretcher and took him back to his room. He was never to leave the hospital again.

The hospital had notified Mr. and Mrs. Hennessey that David was coming back. They were outside his room when I went upstairs. Mr. Hennessey sat on a bench, his head in his hands. Mrs. Hennessey was pacing the corridor. When she saw me, she ran toward me and buried her face in my chest. She was a small woman, with fine features and soft blond hair. David looked a lot like her. Her blue eyes, so much like his, were red from crying. She wasn't crying now, but her face reflected the desperation and sadness of the past months.

She took both my hands in hers. "We thought he was getting better. We thought our prayers had been answered. We were so happy about this weekend—and now he's worse again." She shook her head. "I know it's God's will, but why must there be so much pain for my poor boy? Why?"

I didn't know what to answer her. I never knew what to answer Mrs. Hennessey. I tried to comfort her as best I could, but the words were always meaningless. I realized what I really wanted to do was get out of there, to get as far away from the hospital and David and death and pain as I could.

I made my excuses to Mrs. Hennessey and put my hand on Mr. Hennessey's shoulder as I passed the bench on the way to the elevator. He didn't look up.

I retrieved David's car from the parking lot and just sat in it for a few minutes. I didn't know where I wanted to go. I didn't want to be alone, yet there was no one I wanted to see. Then I thought of Sabrina.

She was sitting in the backyard of the small frame house she shared with her two sons, in Lexington. The boys were away at Scout camp and she was alone. When I walked into the small garden through a space in the privet hedge, it was almost as if she expected me. She put down the book she had been reading, looked up and said, "I've got chili for dinner, want some?"

"Sounds fine." I pulled a green-and-yellow-webbed folding

chair up next to hers and sat down, realizing for the first time how tired and drained I was.

"Didn't go too well with David, huh?"

"How did you know?"

"Well, here it is six o'clock Saturday evening, and you're back. I just put two and two together. But to be honest, I had a feeling it wouldn't. I've been through all that before."

"When?"

"A long time ago, with my mother. I was your age when it happened." She turned and swung one leg over the arm of her chair so that she faced me. She was barefoot and wearing a faded blue tie-dyed caftan, her favorite at-home attire. Her long brown hair was done in a single braid that hung down her back. Usually, she wore it in a ponytail. I kind of liked the braid; it almost made her look exotic, though it was hard to think of Sabrina that way. Her eyes were warm and dark. The kind of eyes that made you think she understood, even if she didn't. She had a good face, strong, high cheekbones and a straight, prominent nose. I had the feeling she was more attractive now than when she was younger. Hers were the sort of looks the owner had to grow into.

"I've been through a lot of shit since then," she went on, "but I think that was the most hideous time of my life. She had cancer too. You get a little nuts when you're living close to terminal illness for any length of time. But you know all about that now, don't you? You question everything—about yourself, about God, about life in general. And then there's the guilt, the awful guilt. How dare you have a good time when your mother is dying? How can you laugh, or go to a movie? And, we all know—sex is out of the question."

"Jesus, Sabrina, are you reading my mind?" I couldn't believe she was articulating everything I had been feeling all day.

"No, I'm not reading your mind. Like I said, I've been there. It's not a unique experience, but once you've had it, you never forget. It leaves a scar right down the middle of your brain. Come on, let's go inside, and I'll fix you a drink. You probably could use one." She got up from her chair and led me into her large kitchen, the most used room in the house. Sabrina loved to cook, and to feed her sons and all of their friends, she had installed a six-burner restaurant stove that took up one whole wall. In the center of the room was a rectangular oak table that could easily seat ten. I had to duck to avoid the ceiling-hung rack that held a large array of pots, pans and kitchen utensils. Charlie, Sabrina's gray Persian cat, was asleep on top of the refrigerator.

"Sit down, Steve." She indicated a chair at the head of the table. "Now what'll you have? Vodka and tonic? Scotch? Beer? You name it, I've got it."

I settled for a beer. She fixed herself a vodka and joined me at the table. I was feeling better. Just being there with Sabrina seemed to help. There were no pressures, nothing to explain; she knew it all. I told her about the day with David, how inadequate I felt, how frightened I was. Then I told her how David wanted me to think about being a doctor. She was on her second vodka. Her elbows were on the table, her head resting in one hand.

"Do you want to be a doctor? You could be if you wanted to."

"That's just it. I don't think I want to. Today in the car, when David was screaming in agony, even if I had been a doctor, there was nothing I could have done to really help him, except give him another shot. At least with the animals we treat, when it comes to it finally, I can put them out of their misery. I couldn't do that for David."

"That's true; but more to the point, are you happy being a vet, or do you want to be a doctor?"

"Maybe I owe it to David to try."

"Christ, Steve!" she said angrily. "You don't owe anything to anyone but yourself. You spend your life pleasing your parents, pleasing Carney, pleasing David. What about Steve? You're a terrific vet. If it makes you happy to help animals—and God knows they need help—then do it!"

She was right, I knew she was right. No way did I really want to be a doctor. I loved caring for animals. There was great satisfaction in making them well and keeping them healthy. I liked the relationships I made with them and with their owners. Perhaps the problem was that I no longer felt my work presented a challenge where I was.

"Maybe it's working for Carney," I said after a moment. "There's got to be more to veterinary medicine than spaying dogs and treating flea infestations."

Sabrina put her glass down, annoyed. "What do you want me to say—there isn't? Of course there is, and no one knows it better than you. Carney's clinic isn't the last bastion of veterinary medicine on earth. Go back to Angell and get your boards in surgery. Go to New York and work for the ASPCA, or that other place, the Animal Medical Center. You've got a hundred options. Take one of them. But whatever it is, do it for you!"

She left the table and went to the stove. A large, black pot of chili had been simmering, circulating luscious smells through the kitchen. Sabrina stirred the pot and brought a spoonful to the table for me to taste. "Need anything? More pepper, maybe?"

"No, it's perfect." I realized how hungry I was. "How come you made so much with the boys away?"

"First of all, I knew you were coming," she said, smiling. "And second, I like to make a big batch and freeze it. Then I'm never unprepared if all of Lexington and Concord come to dinner. See?"

I ended up eating three portions, seriously depleting her stores. We talked until well after midnight, and when I left, I felt almost whole for the first time in months. From time to time, when there was a spare moment at the clinic, Sabrina would quiz me about my plans. I hadn't made any definite decisions, but at least she made me think about it.

I was heading down the hill toward the clinic. It had been a good run. Even at the quickened pace, I wasn't tired. The clinic was almost in sight when it occurred to me. Why *not* New York? I needed to be on my own, away from the support system so generously offered by my family. I needed work more difficult and challenging than what I was doing. Maybe a big-city animal hospital was the ticket.

I slowed down and trotted into Carney's parking lot and unlocked the door of the red Mustang. Before David died, he told me he wanted me to have it. I demurred, but his parents insisted. So now it was mine. It wasn't as shiny as it used to be, but at least I tried to keep it reasonably clean. I took my clothes out of the backseat and went into the clinic to shower and change.

When I had dressed, there was still fifteen minutes until the clinic formally opened. Neither George nor Sabrina had yet arrived. I went to Sabrina's desk, sat down at her typewriter and neatly typed a letter to Dr. Harley Petersen, Director of the ASPCA in New York, asking for a job

Chapter 7

It would be a test. If I could do it—if I could run the twenty-six mile Boston Marathon—that would mean I could go to New York. If I failed to complete the distance, I would take it as a sign and remain in Boston. Undoubtedly, it was an oddball and grueling manner for a supposedly grown-up person to make a life choice. But in those depressing, distracted months after David died, I seemed incapable of finding an easier, more direct way to make the decision.

The answer to my inquiry at the ASPCA had arrived the week before. My hands shook as I opened the envelope and read the reply, offering me an immediate post as a senior staff clinician. God was in his heaven, all was well with the world and I could have the job I dreamed of. The ASPCA was the Peace Corps of veterinary medicine. I would be on the front line, a *real* veterinarian, dealing with animals and people who really needed my help. No more suburban matrons chasing me around the exam table. Finally, I would have the challenge Emily Addison had described when I was fifteen years old.

I should have been elated. Instead, what felt like a cold claw gripped my stomach, and the cold traveled straight to my heart. It was hard to admit, but the very thought of New York scared the hell out of me. New York was where the big stuff happened. It was competitive, it was sophisticated, and even worse, according to some of my friends, it was dangerous. But I was a big boy now and, somehow, I had to prove it. Not to anyone else—to myself. Though my thinking may have been slightly convoluted, at that point the Marathon seemed the ideal trial. It was the race

David had planned to run, and now I would do it—for him, as well as for me.

Along with beans and the Pops, the Marathon is Boston's great claim to fame. Run every Patriots' Day since 1897, the race commemorates Paul Revere's ride on the 18th of April, 1775, to warn the colonists of the approaching British. And for a prize no grander than a bowl of beef stew and a laurel wreath, it attracts the finest runners in the world, as well as thousands of people like me who enter just to be able to say they've done it.

It's estimated that over a million spectators line the twenty-six mile route, which winds through the Massachusetts countryside from the rural hamlet of Hopkinton to the Prudential Center in downtown Boston. They cheer the contestants on with shouts of encouragement and cups of water. For years, I had yelled myself hoarse from the sidelines, filled with admiration for the participants. Fast or slow, young or old, to me every runner was a hero. Now, God help me, I would be one of them.

I decided to tell no one about the letter and the offer at the ASPCA. If I failed to complete the course, I didn't want anybody to know what had been at stake. It would've sounded too silly.

Since I ran almost ten miles every morning, I was already in training of sorts. But when I made my decision to enter, the Marathon was only three weeks away. It was too late for me to qualify by making the mandatory "under three hours" time in another officially sanctioned race. However, there was an odd rule that permitted doctors to run without first qualifying. Figuring that a D.V.M. was close enough to an M.D., I thought I'd chance it as an unofficial entrant, hoping the spotters posted along the route wouldn't notice and pull me ignominiously from the pack the way they did Cathy Switzer in 1967, before women were allowed to enter the event.

For the next three weeks I trained in earnest. Since I had never run more than ten miles at a clip, I could only hope the common wisdom was true—about being able to double whatever distance you ran regularly. Instead, I concentrated on quickening my pace so that, if I did finish, I would at least do it in a respectable time.

"It's the craziest thing I ever heard," my father said when I announced I was entering the race. He shook his head. "Nobody in his right mind would run twenty-six miles. You'll be dead when it's finished, and then what?"

"He won't be dead, he'll have done it!" my sister Marcy piped up defensively. "I think it's super! No one else in this family's ever done anything so exciting!"

"Thank God we've only been blessed with one nut." Knitting his forehead, my father sighed with resignation and returned to his newspaper. Even though he disapproved, he knew once I had made up my mind there was no way I'd be dissuaded.

April 18th dawned cloudy and cool, a perfect day for the race. As the gray light crept through the windows of my tiny apartment in Lexington, I lay in bed for a few extra minutes running the course in my head, picturing the terrain I had carefully noted when I drove the twenty-six miles over and over in my car. I was certain I could go the distance since I had been running an average of sixty-five miles a week for the past three weeks. My only fear was being yanked from the pack by a spotter who might recognize the number on my chest as a handmade phony. I had labored for two hours the night before with white oaktag and a black Magic Marker, painstakingly copying the print size of the official number given to my friend Tom Metcalf, a doctor at Massachusetts General Hospital. Tom was also running without qualifying, though he was doing it legally. His number was 4653. I chose 7777 because seven was lucky, but also because I knew there were about six thousand entrants, and I wanted to be well above that to avoid duplication.

It was not yet 7:00 A.M., when showered, shaved and wearing sweat pants and a warm-up shirt over my running shorts and singlet, I let myself in the kitchen door of my parents' house. My mother, exhibiting a last-minute burst of enthusiasm for my venture, had offered to fix breakfast for me and Tom. He had beaten me there and, seated at the counter, was already halfway through the stack of pancakes before him.

"Sit down. Yours are coming," my mother said, expertly flipping a golden-brown flapjack in the pan. "How many do you want?"

"A lot. As many as you can make." I eyed Tom's plate hungrily.

"They're terrific," Tom said with his mouth full. "Just what we need."

We had pored over every book and article about long-distance running we could find and listened to this advice and that about what to eat before a marathon. The latest theory was stoking up on carbohydrates. Supposedly, they metabolized faster than protein and gave the runner more energy. If true, the enormous stack of pancakes my mother set before me would get me to Boston and back again, with energy to spare.

"Where's Dad?" I asked. By this time, my father usually was up reading his newspaper. I had kind of hoped he'd be here and, by his presence alone, indicate he'd changed his mind about my running. But I guessed that wasn't to be.

"He was so tired last night he decided to sleep a little longer. It's a holiday," my mother said casually. If she was aware anything was amiss, she didn't let it show.

"Let's see your number," Tom said between chomps on his second stack of pancakes.

I carefully unwrapped both numbers—his and mine—from the foil, the only covering I had been able to find, and laid them side by side on the counter. "What do ya think?"

Tom appraised them with a critical eye. "Not bad, not bad at all, and when you're moving, it'll be almost impossible to tell. But lemme ask you something. Why did you pick such a high number? There're only six thousand in the race. Don't you think 7777 is a little obvious?"

Something else for me to worry about. I hadn't thought about that at all, and I didn't want to think about it now. "If they throw me out, they throw me out. Nothing I can do about it!"

"They won't throw you out; they wouldn't dare!" My mother slammed the final stack of pancakes on my plate as if I were one of the officials.

"OK, pal, finish up. We've got to get moving," Tom said, wrapping the numbers in the foil again. "We'll put these on when we get there. Have you got a couple of safety pins, Mrs. Kritsick?"

While my mother rummaged in a drawer for the pins, I devoured the last of the pancakes and washed them down with a glass of milk. It was a breakfast fit for Captain America, but only if Captain America wasn't about to run a marathon. I could barely move. My stomach had become home to what seemed like a fifty-pound lead weight. How could I run twenty-six miles when I could hardly get off the stool? So much for carbohydrate loading.

Tom patted his now rotund belly fondly. "It'll all be gone after the first ten miles," he said with assurance, and he belched loudly.

My mother stuck the pins in my shirt pocket. "If you get tired, please stop. It's not worth killing yourself," she said, echoing my father.

"I will," I promised. I wanted to tell her about the job in New York and why I was running in the first place, but I couldn't. Even she might not understand.

"We'll be watching on TV; wave if you see a camera."

"Don't worry, Mrs. Kritsick, you'll be able to spot him," Tom laughed. "He'll be the one with the phony number."

I had met Tom only a year before, while running my daily Concord–Lexington route. He and his wife had just moved to Concord from Baltimore when he began his residency at Mass. General. Tom was tall and lanky, with the kind of craggy, irregular features that would get better looking as he got older. He was a relative newcomer to running. However, he had taken it up with a vengeance, peppering his speech with the sport's jargon and quoting the exploits and advice of world-class runners like Shorter and Rodgers. It was Frank Shorter who had advised "carbohydrate loading" in an article in *Sports Illustrated*. Tom carried it around in his wallet, pulling it out for reference, like a Born Again Christian with scripture. When we drove into Hopkinton, inching our way behind a mass of stalled and honking traffic, I wondered if Shorter was as stuffed and uncomfortable as I.

The town, an old, upper-middle-class enclave, looked as if it were in the throes of an invasion. But, since the Marathon route has been the same for over seventy years, I assumed the residents were quite used to the jam of cars and the thousands of spectators who lined their neat, perfectly groomed main street every Patriot's Day to watch the start of the race.

It was like a huge carnival. When we arrived, the fifteen-acre tract of land designated a parking area was already filled with what must have been a thousand cars. Spectators and well-wishers milled about offering last-minute encouragement and energy in the form of Hershey bars and orange slices to friends or relatives who were participating in the race. Runners, some still in warm-up clothes, others stripped down to shorts and singlets, supported themselves against cars while they flexed the tension-tightened muscles of their ankles, calves and thighs. Others, legs extended, sat on whatever small piece of ground they could commandeer and stretched, reaching with their hands to the right foot and then the left. Still others jogged nervously in place, the adrenaline coursing prematurely through their veins.

When we had parked the car near a clump of trees at the edge of the tract, I could see some of the entrants were using them as a makeshift lavatory. There weren't enough Johnny-on-the-spots in the field to handle the natural result of the tension and anxiety that beset the runners—the trees had to do.

As we slipped out of our warm-up clothes and locked them in the trunk, a voice with a decided New England twang came through the loudspeaker system and reverberated across the field, calling runners to a starting line that seemed nowhere in sight of the parking lot. Slowly, two by two, in ragtag bunches and singly, people began to move instinctively toward the invisible line, like a great migratory herd. Press helicopters hovered noisily overhead, photographing this human version of lemmings marching to the sea—six thousand people, running for a bowl of beef stew. Maybe my father was right; we were all nuts!

There was still a half hour before the race began. Tom and I picked our patch of ground and stretched our leg muscles carefully for about twenty minutes. There was no sense adding to the eventual discomfort of the run with a pulled Achilles tendon. Then, with great ceremony, I placed the handmade number on the center of my chest and pinned it to my Adidas shirt. I was ready. My heart thumped with anticipation. I could literally feel the adrenaline running in my veins. Suddenly, I too had to make use of that clump of trees.

The better runners and the champions, like Frank Shorter and Bill Rodgers, were way up front wearing low numbers. We joined the rear ranks, a great multicolored mass of men and women jogging in place, stretching to remain warm and limber, or pawing the ground like anxious cattle. The excitement was contagious. An electric kind of camaraderie was transmitted from one runner to the next. We were not unlike an army about to go into battle. I was thrilled to be a part of it, yet at the same time a wave of fear washed over me. What if I tripped and was trampled when the stampede began?

I never heard the starting gun, but a roar came from the crowd up front, and slowly, the pack began to move. My own Boston Marathon had begun. It took a full five minutes before our rank even reached the starting line, over a third of a mile away.

Crowds of cheering people lined both sides of the road that sloped gently downward from Hopkinton. One family had set up a stereo system on their front lawn, and as we passed, the *Star Wars* theme echoed grandly in the cool air. It was fitting background music.

About a mile outside of town, the pack began to thin out, as each runner established his own stride. I looked at my watch. I was running well, shaving a few seconds off my 6:30 training pace. At the start, Tom and I had been shoulder to shoulder, but now I could see the strain in his face. "I've got to slow down," he puffed, "or I'll never make it. Meet you at the Prudential Center." He fell back, and I was on my own, running with strangers, some of whom, during the race, would become comrades.

Energy still high, we sprinted past the rolling Massachusetts farmland, relishing the applause offered by onlookers along the way. Someone yelled, "You're lookin' good 7777." The encouragement so delighted me, I quickened my pace just a fraction.

"Take it easy, kid. You don't want to use it up too fast," the slender gray-haired man running at my side advised. I recognized him from pictures I had seen in the newspapers. He was Tommy Conklin. Now sixty-eight, he had won the Marathon twice: first in the thirties and ten years later in the mid forties. A retired electrician from Cape Cod, he spent his time painting seascapes and running along the beach to train for this race. It was, he told me as he ran with seemingly little effort, his forty-fifth Marathon. Released long ago from having to prove himself by winning, his only objective now was to finish the twenty-six mile course.

With Tommy Conklin pacing me, we made it easily to the first official water station in Framingham, the five-mile mark. Volunteers handed off paper cups filled with water or Gatorade to the passing runners. I grabbed a Gatorade and sipped it for the next fifty yards, careful to keep my hands at chest level to obscure my number from the spotters positioned at each table. The crowd had thickened, and the cheers were louder as we approached the center of town.

"Don't run for *them* now," Tommy cautioned. "Run for yourself. It's the end when you'll need them."

But my body felt good. Running easily, my legs responded to everything I asked of them. Even the weather was cooperating nicely. The temperature had remained a cool 50°, and there was very little wind. If it had been sunny and warm, dehydration would have been a problem, making it necessary to drink more liquid. As it was, body temperature for most of us would increase to at least 102° before the race was over. I couldn't think about that. Now my main concern was getting to Wellesley, the halfway mark.

It was sheer elation that carried me past the 13.1-mile marker, through the lines of cheering Wellesley College girls. If I had died and gone to heaven, it couldn't have been better.

"Sock it to 'em, lucky sevens," a group of them called. "You can do it! You can do it!" another bunch chanted. For one glorious moment, I felt as if I were running all by myself.

"Ain't they somethin'?" Tommy Conklin panted, nudging my arm. "If only I was ten years younger. Finish and that's what you got waitin' for you. They don't care if you win. You're a hero if you just finish."

I checked my watch again. Tommy and I were running the mile in just over six and a half minutes. Not bad for an "unqualified" vet and a retired electrician. The race was half over, and I still had energy to spare. But ahead of us was Newton and the four famous hills, the worst of which was aptly called Heartbreak Hill. It was here the race was made or broken, not only for the lead runners, but for those of us in the pack as well.

At the Wellesley time split, anyone who was running to win picked up his pace, trying to get an edge on the physical effort required to make those awful hills. David had talked endlessly about them, taking it for granted he would be among the front runners. "I have to run the first thirteen miles in under 5:00. Then at Wellesley, I'll break out and, if I can do the stretch before the hills in 4:30, I've got it. Commonwealth Avenue is downhill, so with a final kick, I can finish averaging 4:56 for the course." His eyes shone with determination. "I'm gonna win this damned thing, you can bet on it!"

I would've bet on it. Not because he was my friend, but because he was really good. Before he got sick, David trained daily and twice ran the actual Marathon course, clocking himself at two hours, thirteen minutes, a time good enough for even Shorter and Rodgers.

But David wasn't here, I was. And though I didn't have to concern myself with winning times, I knew at Wellesley, sure as hell, I had to finish this race—for both of us.

Once through Wellesley, the landscape began to change, becoming less rural. Farmhouses and barns gave way to suburban houses, their residents lining the streets, waving, cheering and handing off wet sponges, water and more Gatorade to needy competitors.

The pace quickened, even in the pack, as we ran toward Newton. Everyone in my immediate vicinity seemed to be doing well. Our faces were flushed from exertion, our bodies lathered with sweat, as we pounded the last downhill patch before the four hills. I fixed my attention on the girl directly ahead of me. Tall and lean, with long, supple runner's legs, her blond hair flew out in the wind from beneath the rolled navy bandana tied round her forehead to keep the sweat from her eyes. She wore a navy-blue tank top and white shorts with S E A T emblazoned across her fanny in big block letters. I was admiring S E A T, when suddenly, she tripped, perhaps on a small rock, or a crack in the road, and sprawled headlong in front of me. I darted to the side, and without breaking stride, Tommy Conklin and I each grabbed an arm and helped her to her feet, quickly getting her to the sideline and avoiding a pileup.

Her knee was badly skinned. Pieces of dirt and rock were imbedded in the wound, and she took the bandana from her head and wrapped it around the knee to staunch the blood running down her leg. But hobbling between us to a first-aid station about ten yards down the road, she seemed more angry than hurt. "Goddamn it!" she blurted, "I've been training all year like a Spartan soldier. Now this happens; it's not fair."

"You'll do another," Tommy consoled her. "I've done forty-five of them, there's always next year."

"Yeah, I guess so." She smiled sadly. "You fellows better get back, you'll lose your time. Thanks for helping."

We left her at the station and rejoined the pack. "Good luck!" I heard her yell, and I waved without turning around.

The wind freshened as we ran through Newton Center. Rain had threatened from the start of the race, and now it began to drizzle. The cool mist felt good on my face, giving me an extra boost when I needed it—the first hill was dead ahead. Tommy had taken two orange slices from a helpful spectator, and he handed me one to suck on. "I'm gonna slow down a bit," he said. I could see he was winded. His face had reddened, and the perspiration trickled down his temples from under his white painter's cap. "I'll leave the speed to you young fellas. Like I told you, all I want to do is finish."

"You OK?" I asked, concerned. I liked this sturdy old man I hardly knew.

"Fine. I'm just fine. You go ahead. Nice runnin' with ya, see ya in Boston." He fell back, and I made it up that first hill wondering if I'd be lucky enough to run a marathon when I was sixty-eight.

Now I was really beginning to feel the effects of the distance. The next two hills felt like mountains. My throat was parched, my legs ached and my breath roared in my ears, even louder than the cheers of the thousands of spectators waiting at the approach to Heartbreak Hill.

We were at the twenty-mile mark—only 6.2 miles to go. An extraordinary kind of pain began to shoot through my body, almost as if I were being ripped apart. Every muscle screamed. I wondered if this was what runners called "hitting the wall." When it happens, the agony is so intense, even world-class competitors are forced to drop out. I had to get past it. If I didn't, I'd never be able to finish.

Concentrating on every stride, every footstep, was the key. I couldn't let my mind wander. Up the hill, up the hill. Pound, pound. Don't think about the pain. There is no pain, only asphalt passing beneath my feet. I heard a voice call my name. Was I imagining things? Then again, "Come on, Steve! Do it, do it!" The voice was real. Halfway up the hill, Jody Dougherty, a girl I'd known in high school, appeared at my side with a cup of water and a soaked sponge. I gratefully sipped the water, trying hard not to gulp it in one swig. Jody ran along with me, coaxing and cajoling while I squeezed the sponge over my face and head. "Come on, come on, Steve. Just a little bit more." Her round horn-rimmed glasses slid down her nose, and her bright red hair slipped out of her ponytail and flew around her face as she lured me up the steep incline. If she could've, she would have gotten behind me and shoved. Why, I wondered? I had paid so little attention to her when we were in school, and now, here she was, "The Angel of Heartbreak Hill." Without her, I never would've made it to the top. For a second, I flashed on what unearthly power had sent Jody just when I thought my heart would burst through my chest. I wanted to thank her, but speech was impossible. I could only smile weakly and press her arm.

Then, there it was—Boston! It rose suddenly, like Oz, so close I could almost touch it. The John Hancock building, the Prudential Tower, it was the Emerald City. Now for six more miles the Yellow Brick Road was downhill all the way.

I glanced at Ann, the school teacher from Falmouth, on my right, and the two boys from Italy, on my left. We had been companions ever since Newton, when Tommy Conklin dropped back. Smiles played across their faces, momentarily obscuring the body-breaking agony we shared. They too had seen the city.

Soon, we were running past the brownstone mansions on Beacon Street and into downtown Boston. Push, push! One foot after the other. Only two more miles, a spit. Push! Push! Each leg weighed a hundred pounds, the breath had been sucked from my lungs. Oh God, how I hurt. Push!

The crowds lining both sides of the street were enormous, 30,000, maybe 40,000 people. It could've been Calcutta or Bombay. Behind me, from somewhere in the depth of the mob, a familiar voice screamed, "There goes Steve! Hey, Steve!"

I looked back over my shoulder and saw my sister Charlotte running along the edge of the crowd, waving a Hershey bar. She caught up to me and passed the unwrapped bar of chocolate. I nodded my thanks, shoved two squares in my mouth and gave the rest to Ann and the Italian boys. Chocolate, wonderful gorgeous chocolate. The energy it produced was instant—enough to carry me another half mile. I would have to write the Hershey company about their miraculous product.

The roar of the crowd was deafening as we made the left turn into Boylston Street, providing the final impetus just as Tommy Conklin said it would. It was only five hundred yards to the finish line. A kind of mindless euphoria washed away the pain. Somewhere in a dreamlike distance, I could hear the cheers of the quarter of a million people who formed a sort of human tunnel to the Prudential Center. Ahead of me was the digital time clock, stretched above the finish line, and the officials recording the numbers and yelling out the runners' times. A few more yards, push, push! Another ten feet. Push!

"3:13:47!" the timekeeper called as I crossed the line.

"Slash!" the other official yelled, and brutally ran his black Magic Marker across the handmade number on my chest. I was disqualified. I knew I would be from the start. It wasn't that I was seeking an official sanction. I always knew that was impossible—I was running for me, and no matter what they did, the credit was mine. But now that I had finished the damned race, now that I had run 26.2 miles, I suppose I wanted some small recognition. At the very least, when the man struck me with his black marker he might've said, "I'm sorry." That wasn't too much to ask.

But even the meanness of the finish couldn't diminish the joy I felt as I stumbled down to the Prudential garage to join Bill Rodgers, Frank Shorter and the thousands of other competitors for that legendary bowl of beef stew and all the beer we could drink. Great vats sat on long tables, and volunteers ladled the magic mixture into Styrofoam bowls for the exhausted but happy throng. I was well into my second helping when I spotted Tommy Conklin and then Tom Metcalf, who seemed much wearier than the old man.

I looked around, thrilled to be in such extraordinary company. An emotional high pervaded the cavernous space, attesting to our wondrous achievement. We were a club, a very special club. We had run the Boston Marathon. And having done that, for me at least, anything was possible—even New York. I raised my paper cup of beer in a toast to David. "We did it, buddy. We really did it!"

Chapter 8

The apartment was dark, gloomy and stiflingly hot. The ad in the *New York Times* had read, "Up. E. Side, Air-cond., Cozy Studio, w/bath, kitch., $100." Because the price was right and the apartment was within easy walking distance of the ASPCA, I had taken it on sight, ignoring the fact that in this case, "Up. E. Side" meant the southern border of East Harlem—the ghetto.

The block was noisy and unkempt. Even at eleven in the morning, when I came to see the apartment, many of the street's residents, men as well as women, sat sprawled on the steps of the identical worn brownstones, soaking up the hot June sun. Radios blared from open windows, and the smell of beans and rice cooking pervaded the heavy summer air. Street vendors hawked ice cream and tacos from rolling carts shaded by bright orange-and-black or blue-and-white umbrellas. A fire hydrant had been uncapped, and children, oblivious to the illegality of their pleasure, laughed and splashed in the cool spray that arched into the middle of the street and sent empty cans and scraps of paper rushing through rivulets along the gutter. It was a scene from an old James Cagney movie about New York in the thirties. Only this was 1976, and the characters were Hispanic, not Irish, Italian or Jewish.

But the building itself, though run down, seemed neat and clean. Besides, I imagined living here would give me the feel and texture of the part of the city in which I would work. I thought the apartment would do nicely until I got to know the city better. That, however, was only until my third night in residence, when the much touted "Air-cond." broke down, and complaints to

Mrs. Mercado, the landlady, brought promises but no repairs. "Jaime need to get a part, then he fix right away," she assured me. Jaime was Mrs. Mercado's common-law husband. When he wasn't sitting on the stoop in his undershirt drinking beer and chattering in Spanish to cronies camped around the steps in folding chairs, he was reputed to function as a handyman for the eight apartments in the shabby building. I had yet to see the results of his labor, and since he spoke no English, or pretended not to, talking to him was useless.

Four weeks later, in the midst of the worst July heat wave New York had seen in years, I sleeplessly tossed on the lumpy, pullout bed in my "cozy" studio, bathed in perspiration. The ceaseless beat of Pachanga music pounded through the wall from the apartment next door, and I watched roaches the size of mice dance in tempo up the side of the ancient refrigerator. How dumb I'd been to plunk down three months' rent in advance. "We don' wan' no comers an' goers," Mrs. Mercado had advised me. "Apartments like this one you can't find for no $100. You don' wan' it, I got four guys waitin'—all doctors. People doctors, not like you with animals," she said scornfully. "You wanna palace, you go downtown—for $1,000 a month you get a palace."

In another life Mrs. Mercado probably sold used cars. She convinced me I had no choice but to take the dingy studio since the only alternatives, according to her, were the streets or a Park Avenue penthouse, and I naively believed her. It was too late by the time I realized there were many things more amenable in between. Unless I was willing to forfeit three hundred dollars, she had me. I was stuck on 98th Street with Mrs. Mercado and Jaime for another two months. By then, I would've had my fill of texture.

But I was so pleased with my job at the ASPCA that even the cucarachas and the Pachanga music were tolerable. From the very moment I stepped through the doors of the three-story, red-brick building overlooking the East River at 92nd Street, I was struck by a kind of communal warmth that belied the institution's nondescript, WPA-depression architecture.

The lobby bustled with activity. People and their assorted animals waited at the reception desk to be directed up the long ramp to the clinic. A group of mostly black and Hispanic children laughed and giggled as they toured the facility, taking particular delight in a litter of kittens displayed behind a big picture window. The kittens, recently taken into the shelter, were up for adoption as "the special of the week," and the kids oohed and aahed, their high-pitched voices indicating they wanted them all, while their teacher patiently explained the responsibility involved in caring for an animal.

In a corner alcove, a cheery, middle-aged woman volunteer inveigled any and every passerby to at least look at her charges, fifteen adoptable grown cats, who peered disconsolately from three tiers of cages against the wall. "Wouldn't you like one?" she asked hopefully. "If you take one, spaying or neutering is thrown in free." A bargain hard to resist. When I explained that I was a vet who would be working in the clinic upstairs, she was unfazed. "All the doctors here have at least two of the shelter animals. You'll soon have one, you'll see."

While I was trying to gracefully withdraw from the cat corner, an elderly black man pushed his way through the front door bent under the weight of the sick German shepherd he carried. "Somebody help me," he puffed. "I can't hold him no more!" Before I could reach him, a burly clinic aide ran from behind the desk and relieved the man of his burden, easily carrying the big dog up the ramp in his arms. I followed them to the crowded clinic waiting room, its institutional drabness brightened by a colorful, childlike hand-painted mural of animals that covered the entire back wall.

What I sensed here was vitality and excitement, things I'd rarely felt at George Carney's clinic. In fact, more had happened in the five minutes I had been in this building than took place at George's in a month.

"Glad to see you, Steve. Welcome to Bedlam—animal division!" Harley Petersen, the hospital's director, warmly shook my hand in his scruffy, cluttered office adjoining the clinics. "It's a little frenetic. As usual, we're shorthanded, but you'll get used to it. Anybody who's trained at Angell won't be overwhelmed by what goes on here. Except we have neither the manpower nor the equipment Angell does, so you'll find yourself improvising a lot. Don't worry, you'll pick it up." He smiled broadly.

I liked Harley right away. He was tall and slender, with wavy dark hair going to gray at the temples. His face had the weathered, lined look of the farm in northern New Jersey where he had grown up.

He still lived in Jersey, and though married with three children, the pivot of his life was the hospital, to which he commuted daily. Harley's specialty was orthopedic surgery, and to practice that, there was no better place than the ASPCA. "You want to do orthopedics, you do it on the borderline of the ghetto," he said in the flat accent of his state. "People don't use leashes, and their dogs are constantly being hit by cars. It's not that they don't love their animals, they do. Maybe even more than people with money. It's just that the level of care they can give is generally lower." Harley lit a cigarette and dragged on it deeply. "I've got nine dedicated vets here, ten counting you, and we handle a case load of about 80,000 a year, mostly animals belonging to ethnic minorities. You'll see drunks and drug addicts and people who'll threaten to kill you because they don't have the money to pay for their animal's treatment. You'll see cruelty and abuse, the kind that rarely happens in Lexington, Mass. But a lot of what you'll see is love, plain basic love, and the importance of the relationship between people—especially poor people—and their pets."

He ground out his cigarette and put his arm around my shoulder. "I know you've got the academic credentials, now all you need is a strong heart and an iron constitution. You're not gonna get rich here—no one does—but you'll do good work." He said it with a certainty that made me feel I could and I would. After all, what he described was exactly what I had come to New York for.

In a short time, I fell into the routine of the "A," as everyone who worked there called it, handling twenty-five to thirty cases each long day, beginning at eight in the morning and finishing at eight at night. It was exhausting, but the rewards Harley had promised were immediate. For the first time in two years, I felt I was really practicing veterinary medicine—the kind I had been trained to do at Angell. The hospital was a living laboratory for every possible variety of animal disease and affliction. And, since pets are a relatively accurate reflection of their owners' life-styles and cultures, what I might've previously considered bizarre soon became commonplace.

I had never thought of animals, particularly domestic pets, as having any ethnicity, but they do. Many are treated as members of the family, and like the people with whom they live, they often are what they eat. Chihuahuas, for example, the dog of choice among Hispanic women, are chronically overweight because of steady diets of rice and beans and therefore subject to heart disease and diabetes. The first dog I saw in that condition looked as if it had been blown up with a bicycle pump; its pale skin stretched so tautly over its plump belly, I thought it might split when I palpated the abdomen.

"What do you feed him?" I asked the rotund little Puerto Rican woman, when with great effort she lifted the overstuffed Chihuahua onto the stainless-steel exam table.

"We love him so much, he eat what we eat. Jus' like family, he is," she told me proudly. The family ate some combination of rice and beans at least twice a day, and consequently the dog, lovingly sharing their diet and getting little exercise in the cramped apartment, assumed the proportions of a small pig.

"No more rice and beans for him. If he gains more weight he's gonna die," I explained firmly. "His heart just can't take it. OK?"

"OK, Doctor, whatever you say. We don' wan' nothing should hurt him. He like one of the kids."

Promising to put the Chihuahua on a strict regimen of well-balanced commercial dog food, the woman left. But she would return in several weeks with the dog still weighing in like a prize porker because no one in the family had the heart to deny him his rice and beans.

Still, the overriding factor in dealing with most of our clients was poverty. Even though the fees at the ASPCA were a fraction of those charged by the Animal Medical Center and most private veterinarians, they were still beyond the reach of many people. Often, we were able to improvise with first aid or emergency care for the barest minimum fees, or no cost at all. And there were even those times when an on the spot "by eye" diagnosis was possible, bypassing expensive tests.

One little boy stood tentatively in the doorway of my clinic clutching a small, long-eared dog almost the same chocolate brown color he was. About twelve, the boy was neatly dressed in a Mickey Mouse T-shirt, chino pants and clean white sneakers.

"Come on in," I said gently. His large, wide-set dark eyes flickered with fear, as he tried to push himself over the threshold into the office. "Come on, don't be afraid." I walked across the room and petted the dog he held even tighter in his arms. "That's a cute little dog you've got there. Why don't we put him up on the table so I can really look at him?" I was trying to instill confidence in both of them at the same time. For some kids, going to the vet was as bad as going to the doctor.

"It's a she," he said, reluctantly settling the dog on the exam table. "Her name's Lulu, and I think she has somethin' real bad." His big eyes filled with tears.

I could see from the chart Lulu was a five-year-old mixed breed and the owner's name was Robert Hearns. "Are you Robert?" He nodded, his lower lip quivering. "OK, tell me what you think's the matter."

A tear trickled down his cheek, and his mouth puckered so he wouldn't cry. "I think she's got cancers," he blurted finally. "I been feelin' them for a long time. But I didn't have no money, and my ma said cancer's expensive. So now I've saved up all my lunch money for a month so you can take care of her."

"Cancer! What ever gave you that idea?" I had listened to the dog's heart and lungs and palpated her abdomen. Everything else seemed to be in fine working order, with no sign of disease.

"Up here on her back." Lulu stood patiently while the boy separated her dark hairs to show me what he meant. "I seen all about it on television. They said if you got lumps, that was a sure sign of cancer, and she's got lots of 'em—look!"

I parted the hair further and found a series of small subcutaneous sebaceous cysts that some dogs are prone to. They were benign, and unless they grew to the point where they were cosmetically unsightly, they could remain with the animal for life with no ill effects.

"She doesn't have cancer, Robert," I told him immediately. "Those are just cysts, and unless you're planning to enter Lulu in a beauty contest, we can leave them right where they are. They won't bother her."

His tears turned to a broad, gap-toothed smile. "You sure? You really sure?"

"Positive, absolutely positive!"

He plucked Lulu from the table and smothered her with kisses. "Hey girl, you're not gonna die, ain't that great?" The dog returned his affection, licking his face as if she knew they both had been reprieved. "What do I owe you for the visit, Doc?" he said in a suddenly grown-up, authoritative manner.

I thought about the weeks of anxiety the boy had suffered while he tried to gather enough to pay for what he feared was a major illness. How could I ask him for money? "There'll be no charge. I only looked at her. Didn't do very much. We'll call it a recheck; that's for free."

"You mean it?" He was a little boy again.

"I mean it. Why don't you go and treat yourself to a great big lunch. You deserve it."

The expression of relief and happiness on the kid's face as he literally danced out of the clinic was payment enough. If only all my cases worked out so well.

But I had become used to dealing with unusual and difficult situations rather quickly. Though Harley and my other colleagues were available for backup and consultation, for the most part I was on my own. That became patently clear early one hot, steamy evening in July.

Because of the ten-day heat wave, our case load had increased significantly. Cats were diving out of open windows. Dogs, when they weren't being hit by cars, were carelessly left in them to suffocate. Birds flew out of open cages and kamikazied against walls. Even two turtles were brought in near death because someone had forgotten to fill their bowl on the windowsill after the water

in it had dried up. To add to the mishaps, tempers were short-
ened by the incessant heat, and from my vantage point, the animal population seemed to be bearing the brunt of it.

That afternoon, however, there was a respite from the steady
patient flow. Evidently, unless it was an emergency, no one
wanted to go out on the baking streets. Noting the nearly empty
waiting room, Harley had gone home early, and Sheldon Clarke
had nipped off to make a house call on one of his rich private-
practice clients. Since several vets were on vacation, that left Don
Schwartz in surgery, Diana Cummings and me to handle the few
remaining cases.

Diana, a feline specialist, had come to the A from the University of Colorado. Though she was about thirty-five, there was still
a little-girl look about her. Small and slender, she kept her long
auburn hair tied in a ribbon (a different color every day), and her
warm, wide eyes, almost the same color as her hair, always had a
slightly startled expression. An excellent clinician, Diana had one
great weakness as a vet—she became emotionally involved with
every case, and the irretrievable ones broke her heart. As I understood it, she and her husband, a gynecologist, were now playing
host to eleven cats that had been abandoned either before or after
she treated them.

Diana was dealing with a pair of kittens found half-dead in a
plastic bag in a subway trash bin when Martha Rodriguez
directed the tall, flat-faced man into my clinic. In his arms was an
unconscious, badly bloodied Doberman puppy no more than four
or five months old.

"Ya gotta save my dog, Doctor! Ya gotta do it!" His gray eyes
were red rimmed and watery. His name was Boncek, Richard
Boncek, and when he laid the puppy on the exam table, I
couldn't help but notice the sweet sickening smell of booze that
seemed to come right from the man's pores.

The puppy had severe head trauma and was in deep shock. I
set up an IV rig, placed a catheter in the dog's leg and began administering fluids and steroids. Boncek hovered over me while I
worked, breathing Scotch fumes in my face and slurring his
words. "God, I love that dog—more than anything, more than

my wife!" He rubbed his hands across his chest, trying to get the blood off his dirty blue work shirt.

"If you love him so much, why the hell did you let a puppy like this off the lead in the street?" I said angrily, trying to clean up the small battered head. I was short-tempered too. The city was in a kind of brownout, and the hospital's air conditioners working at half speed did little to cool the building. I was hot, tired and annoyed by the man's apparent negligence. I couldn't be certain if any of the small bones in the skull were broken; we'd have to X-ray. But after a cursory examination, at least I found the dog's limbs and intestines to be intact.

"It didn't happen on the street," Boncek muttered, more to himself than to me. I only half heard him, but something clicked in my head. The sixth sense that had been finely honed in the past few weeks was suddenly activated.

"What do you mean, it didn't happen in the street? Did a truck run through your house?"

"Nah." He didn't look up. "It was just one of those things. It happened, you know how that is. Just get him fixed up, Doc, and I'll get out of here." He shifted his weight impatiently from one foot to the other.

The puppy had come to, whimpering softly. I called for Beau, the clinic aide, to help me get him into X-ray.

"Animals don't come in here looking like this one unless they've been hit by a car. Now you better tell me," I said sharply, "how'd this pup get hurt?"

Boncek was a big man with the musculature of a manual laborer, but I was as big and in much better shape. I glared at him until he knew I meant business. He lowered his head and began to stammer, "Damn dog, goddamned dog, ya know how many times I told him? Ya know how many? At least a million, but he did it anyway."

"Did what?" I prompted him.

"Dumped. Damn dog dumped. Dumped right in the middle of the rug—right in front of me, with me screamin' at him."

"Yeah, so?"

"So he did it one time too many."

"Yeah, so?" I pressed.

"So I picked him up and threw him against the wall. I didn't mean to hurt him so bad. I was mad, I guess. I couldn't help it. I'll never do it again, Doc, I promise. Just fix him up so he'll be all right," he pleaded, "else my wife won't talk to me." He seemed to have no remorse at all.

I looked at the broken ten-pound puppy on the table and then at this two-hundred pound hunk of human debris. Which was really the animal, I wondered? Rage welled up inside me, and the muscle in my jaw started to work. It took all the self-control I could muster not to lift Boncek off his feet and hurl him against the wall, as he had the hapless dog.

Beau came into the room with a rolling stretcher. I helped him transfer the little Doberman from the table, instructed him to take the dog to X-ray and then to Dr. Schwartz in surgery. Meanwhile, I called upstairs to have an ASPCA agent interview Boncek for suspected cruelty. I didn't suspect it, I was certain of it. But this was the routine.

Leaving Boncek waiting in the clinic, I went back to surgery. Don Schwartz was looking at the puppy's X rays.

"He's a little bloody," he said, smiling, "but miraculously unbowed. Luckily, nothing's broken. He'll be running around in a day or two. Car hit him?"

"No, his owner threw him against the wall—new kind of discipline. Don, I don't want to give him back. The guy's a mean drunk. It'll only happen again."

Don sighed deeply. It wasn't the first time he'd seen this sort of thing. "Let the agent handle it, Steve. Don't get involved," he advised. "You can't save everything that comes through here. You'll end up like Diana with a houseful of cats and dogs."

"They'd be company for my roaches," I laughed.

"Listen to me. I'm telling you like a friend. If the agent says it's OK, let the dog go."

Don was probably right. A veteran of fifteen years at the ASPCA, he was no stranger to human cruelty, yet he had none of the cold, aggressive cynicism I usually associated with surgeons. Rumpled and professorial looking, he was one of the best in his field. It was rumored that he had been offered high-paying posts at some of the leading veterinary facilities in the country, but he chose to stay at the A. Some said it was lack of ambition. I preferred to think it was dedication.

"There's lots of guys just dying to work at Angell, or the U. of Pennsylvania," he once told me. "Not everybody wants to work here. It's tough and it's dirty. But I know I'm really needed. Poor people love their animals as much as rich ones, and when I put my head on the pillow at night and know I've helped them—it makes me feel good."

I took the puppy back to the treatment room, made certain he was put in a cage under heat lamps and left him in Beau's care. With nothing broken, the problem was concussion and shock. We would continue giving him fluids and antibiotics for the next twenty-four hours, until he was up and around. He was a good-looking little dog, black, with tan points on his ears, muzzle and tail. His ears had yet to be docked in the prescribed Doberman fashion, so they flopped down, giving his still unformed baby face an even more innocent cast. It was hard to believe anyone could willfully hurt him.

Walter Schroeder, the cruelty agent, had finished interviewing Boncek when I returned to the clinic. He buttonholed me outside the door and whispered as if he were passing secret plans. "The fella's really sorry, says it'll never happen again." He gestured at Boncek with his head. "Says he loves the dog more than his wife. What more can we ask? I'm not gonna file charges; I think he should have the dog back." Schroeder was a short stocky man with gentle brown eyes. I suppose he had seen much worse than a puppy thrown against a wall in his twenty years on the job. But still, it was hard for me to accept his verdict.

I didn't answer for a moment, wondering how Boncek must treat his wife and looking for a viable way out for the dog and for me. Then, as if someone else were speaking, I heard myself say, "That's too bad. The puppy has such severe head trauma, we think there might be brain damage." I took a deep breath. "The only humane course we can recommend is putting the dog to sleep." Once it was out—it was out. I had never done that before, lied about a patient. Not this way. But I was certain Boncek would act up again, and next time the puppy might not survive.

"Whatever you fellows think." Schroeder was still whispering. "But we'll have to get him to sign a release."

Boncek's face was expressionless when I repeated what I had told Walter Schroeder. He signed the release giving us permission to put the dog to sleep with what I thought was an attitude of relief. Then as he reached the door, he suddenly wheeled on us. "You sons of bitches could've saved him!" he screamed. "Just because I'm not some nigger, or spic, what's mine ain't important to you!"

"That's not true, Mr. Boncek," I said quietly. "What's important to us is the dog and doing what's best for him. Remember, it was you who threw him against the wall and bashed his head in."

He glared at me with wildly darting glassy eyes, clenching and unclenching his fists for maybe about thirty seconds. Then, without another word, he spun around and stalked out. Perhaps he knew if he stayed longer he would display the same uncontrolled violence that had hurt the puppy.

"It's the heat," Schroeder said, shrugging his shoulders. "Makes people nuts."

"Heat, hell," I shot back at him. "He's no better in January than he is in July. You can bet on it."

I had done the right thing, lie or no lie. I was sure of that now. What remained was to find a good home for my new charge.

In the treatment room, Diana was setting up IV rigs for the two calico kittens, who lay head to head in a large cage. "That woman found them in the nick of time." She secured a catheter to one kitten's leg with a piece of tape. "Another hour, they'd've been goners. But we'll plump them up and, in a week or so, put them out for adoption. I'd take them myself, but Todd says one more cat and we call the lawyers," she laughed.

Down the line, in a smaller cage, the Doberman pup lay listlessly on his side. I listened to his heart, checked his gums, which had gotten pinker since we began treatment. I adjusted the catheter through which flowed the life-strengthening fluids. "That's a good fella," I soothed him. "You're gonna be OK now. We'll see to that."

"I heard what happened to him, poor thing. That bastard doesn't deserve him," Diana said vehemently.

"He's not gonna have him."

"I thought Schroeder said it was OK?"

"He did. But I told him the dog was too far gone, we had to put him to sleep."

"Is he?"

"Of course not. Look at him."

Diana opened the cage and tenderly petted the puppy, at the same time appraising his condition. "He's badly beat up, but I think you're right. He'll pull through fine." Her hand trailed over the dog's small form. "He's beautiful, Steve, just beautiful." She looked up at me, pausing for a moment, as if she were seeing me for the first time. "You know, what you did was terrific, just terrific. I was wrong about you."

"How do you mean?" I was surprised that she thought about me at all.

"Well, when I first met you, you seemed so straight arrow, squeaky clean. I said to myself, 'Now there's a guy who goes by the book. Sweet—but always according to the rules.'" She half smiled and little lines crinkled around her auburn eyes. "But you don't always, do you?"

I didn't know whether to be offended or complimented. "Not when it's something like this, I don't. I've been known to bend a rule or two for my own ends, or maybe even for someone else's." I hated the idea that she thought I was a Boy Scout. "I must make a lousy first impression."

"Not at all," she countered. "Like I said, I thought you were sweet—"

"That is the worst word. It sounds like treacle candy."

"I meant it in the best way. But it doesn't matter, because now I think you're much more than that. You did good, Steve, real good!" She stood up and put both her hands on mine. "I'm very pleased you're working with us. I really am." She smiled warmly, and I knew she meant it.

"OK, now that's settled, you have to help me find a good home for him."

"Consider it done. He's a purebred, it'll be easy enough." She thought for a moment. "Matter of fact, we have some friends in Connecticut who just lost their dog. I'm gonna call them as soon as I finish here." She looked once again at the kittens she had dubbed Marie and Antoinette and instructed Beau to watch over them, since he would be on duty all night.

"OK, finito! I'm getting out of here. God, I'm tired," she groaned, leaning over and holding her back. "It's been the most miserable day. I'm going home and sit in the tub for at least three hours. What're you gonna do?"

We ambled down the long corridor back to the clinics. "I don't know, maybe I'll go to a movie. My air conditioner's broken. Can't go home till it cools off outside." I wasn't looking forward to another night in Mrs. Mercado's rental oven. The day I was out of that dump couldn't come too soon.

"That's too bad. I'd ask you to come home with me, but Todd's mother's staying with us. Whatever you do, have fun!" Diana instructed. "I'll call my friends about the pup and let you know." She ducked into her clinic and I turned into mine immediately next door.

I sat on the battered rolltop desk near the window watching the lights twink on in apartment buildings across the East River in Queens. Cars whizzed by on the drive below, headed for what I was certain were definite and cool destinations. I had no destination, nothing to do and no one to do it with. For the first time since I had come to New York, I was lonely. I knew a few people here, but none I wanted to call, even to go to a movie.

"Steve, my boy, I've been looking for you." I turned and saw Dr. Sheldon Clarke standing in the doorway with his hands on his hips. "Thought you might like to go to a bon voyage party on the QE2 this evening," he said cheerily.

The QE2! Was I dreaming? The cherubic little man had appeared like an answer to a subconscious prayer. "I'd love to," I said quickly before he went up in a puff of smoke or changed his mind. The *QE2* was such a delightful alternative to the hot, dull evening looming before me, I didn't even bother to ask who was sailing. I would've been pleased to wish Attila the Hun a safe crossing.

Sheldon Clarke was a legend, not only at the ASPCA, but throughout the veterinary profession. He was seventy-four years old, though nothing in his demeanor, bearing or dress betrayed his years. His energy was boundless. Working longer hours than most of his younger colleagues, he was always perfectly turned out, his shirts and ties carefully chosen to match his jackets or suits. Now, for example, he wore a light-blue shirt, a pale-blue and peach striped cotton tie and a navy gold-buttoned blazer, all calculated to set off the twinkly blue eyes behind his rimless glasses.

Dr. Clarke had been a fixture at the A for over twenty-five years. At the same time, he maintained a lucrative private practice catering to theatrical celebrities and a seemingly endless stream of rich foreigners.

For some reason he had taken a shine to me from the very first moment we were introduced. Whenever possible, he would take me with him when he made evening house calls, presenting me to his clients like a son who might inherit the business. I loved it. Not only did I enjoy the older man's elfin good company, but it gave me the rare opportunity to see how the other half lived, a pleasant respite from the roaches on 98th Street and my usual client roster at the clinic.

I would have to change from the T-shirt and jeans I wore under my lab coat. I arranged to meet Dr. Clarke in front of the building in half an hour. He had his car, and we would drive down to Pier 15 at West 54th Street on the Hudson River. As I was leaving, Diana stuck her head out of her office, all smiles. "Whenever your Dobie's ready, he's got ten acres in Connecticut. My friends would love to have him."

"That's great, Diana. One less to worry about. Guess what? Sheldon Clarke's taking me to a bon voyage party on the *QE2* tonight. Looks like me and my pup both struck it rich!"

"Hey, that sounds like fun. I'll trade you my mother-in-law and my bathtub," she laughed. "Who's sailing?"

"I don't know. One of his fancy clients, I guess. I didn't ask."

Showered and changed from the jeans and sweaty T-shirt to a fresh shirt, tie and light flannel slacks, my jacket over my arm, I walked the six steamy blocks from my studio back to the A. Dr. Clarke waited, leaning against his 1972 beige Volvo sedan. It was almost nine o'clock. Darkness had fallen on the city, but waves of heat still rose from the pavement. The streets around the hospital were as alive and crowded as they might've been at midday.

Not everyone in New York has an air conditioner. Many choose the questionable comfort of the sidewalks over their unbearably stuffy apartments. They cluster in groups around lamp posts, or on camp chairs in front of buildings. Some set up card tables, and the men play quiet, intense games of pinochle or dominos, while the women laugh and gossip on the steps nearby, rocking babies in strollers or cradling dozing older children in their arms. Heat is no longer the great class equalizer—air conditioning has seen to that. Suffering through the summer is now pretty much the province of the poor.

Sheldon Clarke zipped through Central Park at 96th Street, across town to the West Side Highway, barely avoiding a collision with a taxi at Amsterdam Avenue and almost running down a jogger crossing West End. It wasn't that he didn't see well; his eyesight was remarkably good for a man his age, as he was quick to point out. The problem was one of inattention. Dr. Clarke was a terrifying driver. He was the kind who turned his head to look at his passenger when he spoke, completely ignoring what was going on in front of him and cursing the incompetence of others on the road as they desperately swerved to avoid him.

My knuckles white from clutching the door handle, my foot practically through the floor as I stepped on an imaginary brake, I listened as Dr. Clarke explained about Princess Farah Naz and her pigeon, Pierre. It was they we would wave to as the *QE2* slipped her moorings and sailed on the midnight tide.

Pierre was an ordinary New York City street pigeon who lucked

out when the princess's chauffeur struck him as he pulled her
limousine into a parking spot. Farah Naz, it seemed, was a bird
fancier. She leaped from the car, gathered up the injured bird and
immediately called Dr. Clarke, who had attended some of her
other animals.

The pigeon had sustained a bad case of shock as well as a shattered wing. Dr. Clarke treated him, and he recovered splendidly,
except he was unable to fly. Dubbing him Pierre, Farah Naz
adopted the bird, and he remained with her in her Beekman
Place townhouse, soon becoming her constant companion. That
was two years ago. She took the pigeon everywhere with her, and
since she had decided it would depress him to fly vicariously,
twice yearly she booked passage for them both on the *QE2*. In
winter they went to her chalet in Gstaad and in summer to a villa
she kept near Cap d'Antibes. Spring and fall were passed in New
York. According to Sheldon Clarke, Pierre traveled in a specially
designed Gucci carrier. Not a bad life, I thought—even if you
weren't a pigeon.

"She's Iranian, or one of those things," Dr. Clarke told me, as
we turned off the highway ramp at 54th Street. "I've been taking
care of her pets for years. The Duchess of Windsor recommended
me to her. I used to take care of her dogs, hers and the Duke's,
when they stayed here at the Waldorf—they had pugs, you know.
Very nice people. Loved those dogs, they did."

I reflexively put my hand over my eyes when he seemed headed
directly for a series of metal stanchions under the highway. He
noticed my anxiety. Annoyed, he said, "You're as bad as my wife.
Don't worry, I'm a very good driver. Haven't had an accident in
forty-five years, not gonna have one now." He drove the car between the stanchions like a slalom racer and swung into the parking lot alongside the pier.

When I removed my hand from my eyes, I looked up and saw
it—a white ship the size of a mountain, ablaze with light from its
portholes and the string of small dress lights stretched in an arc
over its funnels from bow to stern. The closest I had ever come to
an ocean liner was the movie that was always on television with
Barbara Stanwyck and Clifton Webb about the sinking of the *Ti-*

tanic. But there was no way a movie could approximate the real thing. The *QE2* was as long as a city block and as high as a five-story apartment building. I was truly awed.

"Have you ever sailed on one of these?" I asked Dr. Clarke.

"Really something, isn't she. But I'll tell you, she's not half as grand as the old *Queen Mary.* Now there was a ship. My wife and I sailed on her right after the war. Went to England, we did. I'd been there with the K-9 Corps during the invasion of Normandy. Went over on a troop ship—crowded—awful. I vowed if I survived, I'd go again with Helena—that's my wife—the right way, and we did. None of this polyester and plastic. The *Mary* had solid mahogany furniture and oriental rugs in the staterooms. The service was like the finest hotel in the world and the food—" He bunched his lips and brought his fingers up to his mouth as if he were blowing a kiss. "I think about it, and my mouth waters. My boy, you missed a great time. It's all over now, the great ships. This is all that's left. Not bad, I'll admit, but not the same."

He was muttering to himself, "Not the same, not the same at all," as we strode up the gangplank. An officer in white uniform, with gold epaulets on his shoulders, greeted us at the top. "Visitors or passengers?" he inquired in a clipped English accent.

"Visitors," Dr. Clarke answered. "We're seeing off the Princess Farah Naz."

"Your names, sir?"

"Clarke, Dr. Sheldon Clarke and friend."

The officer glanced down a list of typewritten names attached to a clipboard. "Ah yes, Dr. Clarke. And your friend's name?" He looked at me, raising an eyebrow.

"Kritsick, Dr. Stephen Kritsick. He won't be on your list, he's my guest," Dr. Clarke told him.

"I'm afraid I'll have to check that, sir. We can't be too careful these days." The officer sounded like a particularly snobbish headwaiter.

"The princess told me I could bring anyone I liked. We've never had a problem before." Sheldon Clarke was plainly annoyed.

"I'm certain she did, sir, but I must check it this time. We can't allow just anybody on board without authorization." He picked up the phone at the head of the gangway and dialed, while we stood by uncomfortably, holding up the line of visitors and passengers waiting to board.

"Do you spell that Kripsick with a *K*, or a *C*?" he asked officiously, his hand over the mouthpiece.

"With a *K*, and it's *Kritsick!*" I wondered if I looked like a potential stowaway, or maybe even a terrorist. Well, if it came to it, I could always catch a bus back to 96th Street and then take the crosstown home to the sweatbox. My romance with the *QE2* might be briefer than I supposed.

Finally, after speaking a few words we couldn't hear into the phone, the officer looked up stiffly. "The princess is expecting you both. Sorry about the delay, sir," he said to me.

"Perfectly all right. You just can't be too careful." I mimicked him with all the delight of a successful gate-crasher, but he was not amused.

"The Princess Farah Naz is in the Queen Elizabeth Suite, on the Signal Deck. Take the companionway to your right or the elevator," he directed.

The Signal Deck was at the very top of the ship. We could've taken the elevator, but Dr. Clarke wanted me to have the ten-cent tour of the liner. We made our way up the stairs to the Promenade Deck through gaggles of slightly tipsy departing voyagers and their guests, past a jangle of porters with wagonloads of luggage, and white-coated stewards carrying enormous baskets of cellophane-wrapped fruit and bouquets of flowers. Waiters with trays of champagne seemed to be everywhere.

"There's still nothing like sailing. Most civilized way to travel," Sheldon Clarke pronounced, as he hurried me along a red-carpeted passageway. Some of the stateroom doors were ajar, and the sounds of laughter and ice clinking in glasses floated through the air around us. Who were all these people lucky enough to afford such a trip? They were "other" people, I thought. The ones who lived in the elegant, high-ceilinged, book-lined rooms I saw from the street when I walked the blocks between Fifth Avenue and

Lexington Avenue in the 60s and 70s. I wondered if I would ever be one of those "other" people. Right now, it seemed so unattainable.

Little beads of perspiration had appeared on Dr. Clarke's domed forehead. He patted them with a neatly pressed handkerchief taken from his hip pocket, careful not to disturb the few strands of gray hair strategically placed across the top of his head.

"Take a look in here, Steve." He steered me through a huge set of double doors into an enormous chandeliered room where a full orchestra in black tie was playing a medley of Beatles music. Their audience, four little girls about ten, energetically danced on the parquet floor. "This is the Queen's Room. Not bad, but nothing like the Grand Saloon on the *Mary*. That was real elegance, all crystal and mahogany. Now they have Las Vegas floor shows. What can you do? Nothing stays the same." The old man sighed and pulled me across the cavernous room to a door on the other side of the orchestra. "We can get to the Signal Deck through here." He seemed to know the ship as well as anyone who had made several crossings on her. "I should," he told me. "I've seen the princess and that bird off four times."

There were eight deluxe suites on the Signal Deck. The Queen Elizabeth Suite was the largest and most luxurious. "Costs her over fifteen thousand just to go one way, would you believe that?" Dr. Clarke shook his head. "And that doesn't include the bird—forty dollars extra for the pigeon. You'd think they'd let him ride for free."

I couldn't believe it. That was almost as much as I made in a year. Farah Naz was somehow related to the Shah of Iran—an aunt, or a cousin—Dr. Clarke was kind of vague about it. "Oil," he said. "That's what it all comes from—oil! We're paying for this suite at the gas pump. But with a little bad there's always a little good. She's very generous with her donations to the A. Gave us $25,000 last year. With luck I think I may be able to get a little more this year, so be extra nice. It's not for nothing I wave good-bye to that pigeon twice a year."

A white-coated butler answered our knock at the door of the Queen Elizabeth Suite. "Good evening, Dr. Clarke, Dr. Kritsick." He bowed slightly. He must have gotten my name from the prissy officer at the gangway.

"Good evening, Ahmed. Got your pills this time?" Dr. Clarke inquired familiarly.

"Ah yes, Dr. Clarke, sir. I will not be ill this voyage. I have already taken them. I thank you for asking after my health. Her highness is expecting you. Please come this way." His English was heavily accented, but good. He bowed even lower and, with one arm extended, led us through the long foyer into a double-height living room that was furnished in a style I would've expected to find in an English country home rather than a ship's stateroom. However, since I had been in neither, it was hard for me to judge. And as I later discovered, this was no ordinary stateroom, or suite for that matter. It was a duplex apartment with three bedrooms, a sitting room, two baths and a veranda upstairs; and downstairs, a dining room, kitchen, servants' quarters and the large, comfortable living room with French doors leading to a terrace. I suppose the princess was getting her money's worth.

The room was crowded with well-dressed people speaking a variety of languages and sipping champagne from fluted crystal glasses belonging to Farah Naz. Dr. Clarke told me the princess always brought her own crystal and silver when she traveled. A white-gloved, white-jacketed waiter silently circulated through the crowd, offering a tray laden with a large silver bowl on a bed of ice. The bowl was filled with glittering black caviar. When he approached us, Dr. Clarke whispered, "Have some. It's from the Shah's private preserve."

"I hate caviar," I whispered back.

"Try it," he insisted. "How many times in your life will you have a chance to eat the Shah's caviar?"

I reluctantly spooned the tiny black eggs on a sliver of trimmed toast.

"Put some egg and onion on it," Dr. Clarke coached. "It's better that way." He helped himself from the two small silver bowls next to the caviar, neatly piling the chopped hard-boiled egg and onion onto the Shah's best, and slipped the morsel into his mouth. The expression on his face was one of sheer ecstasy as his cheeks puffed out and he crunched on what he had explained was one of the world's great delights. "Go on, try it," he said, his mouth still full.

While the waiter patiently stood by, I laid the egg and onion on and popped the concoction in my mouth, prepared for the worst. But the taste was extraordinary, nothing like that awful fishy gunk served at weddings and class reunions. I let it roll around in my mouth, savoring the combination of egg, onion and that remarkable black stuff. I was about to reach for more, but our waiter had drifted off, to be replaced by another white-gloved man proffering glasses of champagne from a huge silver tray. I took one and washed down the remnants of the caviar.

"Well?" Dr. Clarke asked smugly, as if he'd invented it all.

"It's great, really great! Why didn't I know about this before?"

"You hang around with the wrong people," the old man laughed.

For a moment, I thought about Mrs. Mercado and Jaime, but only for a moment. Because, suddenly, the crowd parted and she was there. I had never seen anyone quite like her before, at least not in real life. The Princess Farah Naz was somewhere around sixty and not a beautiful woman by anyone's standards. She was tiny and very dark, almost swarthy, with a prominent hawkish nose, deep-set brown-black eyes and coal black hair that looked as if it might have been touched up so the gray wouldn't show. She was wearing a full-length peacock blue gown, embroidered with gold thread around the sleeves and down the sides. Around her throat was a necklace of diamonds and emeralds, and her left hand was weighted down with a matching bracelet. Two diamond-encrusted combs held her dark hair in place on either side of her head. Perched on her shoulder, oblivious to the splendor around him, was Pierre, the New York street pigeon.

"My dear Dr. Clarke, how good of you to come see us off," the princess said in a smoky voice, her English barely accented. "And this is your associate, Dr. Kritsick?" She reached for my right hand to shake it, and I quickly switched the champagne to my left, hoping she wouldn't feel the dampness from the glass. "You didn't tell me he was so handsome. Perhaps Pierre will have to change vets," she laughed.

I felt the blood rush up past my collar to my ears. She didn't let go of my hand, and I glanced helplessly at Dr. Clarke, who seemed amused.

"No, no, dear Dr. Clarke. I'm only joking." She put her slender bejeweled hand on Sheldon Clarke's arm to reassure him.

"I certainly hope so. Pierre's my favorite rags-to-riches patient. Though I will say, in a pinch, you wouldn't do badly with our young friend here." Dr. Clarke smiled at me like a doting parent.

The princess moved on to her other guests, and Dr. Clarke and I sidled up to the waiter with the caviar. I'm not quite sure how it happened, but suddenly there was a great clatter that sounded like a tray with all the private crystal had dropped. There were shouts from the other end of the room near the open French doors. "He's gone!" I heard the princess yell. "Someone help me, quickly!"

Dr. Clarke and I made our way across the room and found Farah Naz and several guests out on the terrace, looking up toward the top of the Signal Deck. Though it was dark, the dress lights, like a string of illuminated diamonds, provided enough light to fully outline the upper decks.

"It must have been the noise. All that crashing frightened him, and he flew out the doors. I never should have left them open," the princess said when she saw us, with no evident concern for her smashed crystal.

"I thought you told me he couldn't fly," I said to Dr. Clarke.

"He can't, but he can kind of flutter, and I guess that's what he did."

Farah Naz was wringing her hands. "This ship can't sail until we find him. You have to help me find him."

"We will, don't worry. He can't have gotten very far," Sheldon Clarke soothed her.

I leaned over the terrace railing and looked below to the Quarterdeck. There, perched on the rail calmly admiring the view of New Jersey, was Pierre. "I see him!" I announced. "I'll get him."

I ran out of the suite and found the outside stairs to the Quarter-deck. The princess followed me and we both clattered down the steep varnished steps, almost landing in a heap at the bottom.

"Shhh!" I put my finger to my lips. "Let's try not to frighten him any more. I'll just come up from behind and grab him."

"Don't hurt him," she whispered.

"I won't." I motioned her away and crept toward the rail, edging closer to the pigeon. Luckily, there was no one else on the deck. A sudden noise might startle him, and he would topple to the Promenade Deck, fifty feet below. I reached up slowly, moving my fingers along the rail, encircled the bird with one hand and quickly pulled him to my chest, amidst a great squawking and fluttering of wings. "Gotchya, my little friend. No more short hops for you," I told him, handing him over to the princess. "There you are, Your Highness, Lucky Pierre, the pigeon with more lives than any pigeon has a right to. I think you'd better keep him in a cage or leave the terrace doors closed for the rest of the trip."

"I suppose I must do one or the other." She stroked the bird's head. "I don't understand it; he's never flown before."

"Well, now that he's done it, he may decide he likes it, so be careful."

She reached up and touched my cheek. "I can't thank you enough. You're a very wonderful young man, very wonderful." She clutched the perfectly ordinary gray pigeon to her bosom as if he were the Maltese Falcon and slowly climbed the stairs back to her suite.

"This is a most remarkable fellow," she told a beaming Dr. Clarke. "Most remarkable. He saved Pierre, just as you did. I want to do something for him," she said, impetuously turning to me. "What would you like? Name it."

I felt my face redden again. I was pleased to have been able to help. I wanted nothing in return; I told her that.

"There must be something you'd like," she insisted. "Every-one wants something."

Wondrous thoughts flew into my head. An apartment with an air conditioner—no, make it one with high ceilings, lined with books—or maybe a new car. I'd had to leave the Mustang home when I came to New York because I couldn't afford a garage, so it had better be a car with a garage. And while we're at it—how about a trip on the QE2? Any or all of the above would do fine, thank you. But I couldn't and didn't wish to ask for anything. Yet I knew she would press until I did. Then it came to me. I thought it would please her, and it would delight me. "You don't suppose I might have some of that caviar to take home?" I asked tentatively.

"That's all you want?" she laughed. "It's not enough, but of course you shall have it." She called Ahmed and gave him instructions.

"I thought you hated caviar." Dr. Clarke smiled smugly.

"I do, I mean I did—until tonight."

Ahmed appeared with a neatly wrapped package. Farah Naz took it from him and handed it to me. "Don't eat it all at once, you'll get sick," she warned. "When we return, Pierre and I look forward to seeing you both." She took my hand, but spoke to Dr. Clarke. "He's a very remarkable young man, dear Dr. Clarke, very remarkable," she repeated. I could swear I saw her wink at him.

Later that night, I sat on my lumpy bed watching Cary Grant and Katharine Hepburn in *The Philadelphia Story* on the new little TV set I had just bought. The air conditioner still didn't work, and the Pachanga music pounded through the wall, competing with the movie. But in my lap, on a tray I had fashioned from a folded *New York Times,* was a full pint of the Shah's caviar. It rested in a soup bowl filled with ice I had chipped with a screwdriver. Alongside were two small dishes of chopped onion and hard-boiled egg. I neatly layered the combination on a Triscuit, popped it in my mouth and wished I had a little champagne to toast the Princess Farah Naz and the QE2. Someday, maybe—someday.

Chapter 9

"DOCTOR KRITSICK, EMERGENCY! DOCTOR KRITSICK, EMER-GENCY BOOTH 3!"

Damn! I had just taken the first bite of a pizza Kenny Gilbert had stowed behind the EKG machine in the cardiology clinic. I hadn't eaten all day, and my stomach was making noises so loud the last dog I examined barked at it. I took one more bite and put the half-eaten slice back in the carton, knowing full well it would be gone when I returned. The AMC cafeteria closed at 3:00, and after that we were on our own, depending on the balky vending machine and whatever junk food was spirited in for sustenance.

Chewing as fast as I could, I ran down the corridor to Booth 3 and swallowed the last chunk of pizza before entering. It was Jim Hartley again, looking as nervous and undone as when I'd last seen him. His lank brown hair was plastered to his head with perspiration and his horn-rimmed glasses slid down his nose.

"What've you got there, Jim?"

"An HBC, Steve. He's pretty shocky. Temperature's 99 and he's got a thready pulse. I just thought you should— I mean—"

"I know, you thought I should have a look before you began treatment," I finished for him.

"Yeah, I mean he's bleeding so badly."

Hartley was right. There was blood everywhere, on the table, on the floor and all over the front of Hartley's white lab coat. The dog, a black and white Lhasa Apso was bleeding from the nose and mouth. He was covered with a blood-soaked woman's jacket.

The owner of the jacket and of the dog stood nearby, trying not to cry. In spite of it all, the dog was still conscious.

"What's his name?" I asked her.

"Harry, his name's Harry, and it's all my fault. I'm so sorry. I never should've let him off the lead."

I handed her the jacket, and she clutched it to her chest. She was young, no more than thirty, well dressed and very attractive. Her dark brown hair was cut short and curled softly around her face. Her hazel eyes were filled with tears.

"OK, Harry, let's see how bad this really is." I lifted the Lhasa's lip and pressed against the mucous membrane. The color was good. Several teeth had been knocked out, causing most of the blood in the mouth. I palpated his abdomen. The liver, spleen and bladder all seemed to be intact.

"Jim, get some epinephrine packs and call a clinic aide in here with a cart."

Hartley yelled down the corridor for an aide and pulled the packs from a cabinet in the booth. While I flexed and extended the dog's limbs to check for broken bones, Jim pushed the small swab packs up its nostrils to staunch the blood.

"I think you may be lucky," I told the woman. "It looks worse than it really is. We'll take him back and get some fluids into him for the shock and take some X rays, though I don't think anything's broken."

"Oh, thank God!" She dropped the jacket and threw her arms around me. She smelled terrific.

I reluctantly disentangled myself from her. "But he's not out of the woods yet," I warned. "With an HBC, particularly when there's head trauma, they're not completely out of danger for at least twelve hours."

She leaned over the table and kissed the dog's bloody face. "I'm sorry, Harry, really sorry. Please be all right—please!"

"He's got a real good chance," I told her, as we carefully transferred the dog to the rolling stretcher Tyler had brought in. "Why don't you wait outside, Miss—?"

"Walker, Andrea Walker; it's on Harry's chart."

"OK, Miss Walker. I'll be back in about fifteen minutes to talk with you. Make yourself comfortable and try not to worry too much."

"One question before you go, Doctor—what *is* an HBC?"

"Hit by car," I explained quickly, as we rolled the stretcher out of the booth and down the long corridor to the surgery prep room.

Hartley, his wooden clogs clopping, ran alongside the table. "Not bad, huh?"

"Not good, but I think he'll make it."

"Not the dog, Steve—her! She's a knockout. I should've handled this one myself," he panted.

"You should've. Maybe next time you won't be so quick to call me. You really ought to try things on your own. I'll help you if you get stuck, but at least start the procedures." I said it, but I knew it wouldn't help. I had made excuses for him before, but he was just hopeless. Hartley was incapable of making a fast medical decision. He was not the guy I'd pick to be with when World War III began.

The prep room was bustling when we rolled in. Three of the five treatment tables were already occupied. Kate Gilchrist was catheterizing a screaming cat with a blocked urethra. Jonas was cleaning and clipping a dog who'd been in a fight, and Barbara, the ward nurse, was giving IV fluids to a post-op kitten. We laid Harry on a vacant table. The bleeding from the nose had stopped, but the hair around his muzzle and long, floppy ears was matted with blood.

"I've got an HBC here! Needs IV fluids and steroids, quick! Where's Susan?" I called for the other surgical nurse.

"Right here, Steve." She rounded the corner and picked up the IV rig and the fluids all in one motion. I inserted the catheter into Harry's jugular vein, and Susan attached the IV tube to it. In seconds, lactated Ringer's solution was flowing through the dog's veins. I instructed Hartley to get some steroids into him, while I pinched the pads of the Lhasa's paws with a hemostat to check his pain reflexes. Harry whimpered when I did it.

"It's all right, fella. I'm not gonna hurt you." The dog looked at me balefully with his almond-shaped Lhasa eyes.

"Susan, let's get a urinary catheter in. I want to see if there's any blood. The bladder seemed all right when I palpated, but we need to make sure. Then clean him up."

Hartley held him while Susan inserted a slender tube into the dog's penis. The other end of the tube was attached to a syringe. She slowly pulled back on the plunger, and clear yellow liquid ran up the transparent plastic tube. In the bladder department at least, Harry was home free.

Kenny Gilbert burst through the double doors of the prep room with an enormous calico cat laid out on a rolling stretcher. He was so excited, his curly yellow hair seemed electrified. "I've got the record, I know I do! High rise—twenty-two stories—and would you believe the son of a gun only has a fractured pelvis, a couple of broken ribs and a pneumothorax? Have him fixed up in no time. Then I've won the pool. How much is in it now, fifty bucks would you say?" Kenny set up the IV rig and inserted a jugular catheter in the cat's neck.

"Damn!" Kate raised her head from her howling patient. "I thought I had it last week with fifteen stories. Are you sure it's twenty-two? You're not embroidering just a little, Kenny?"

"Me embroider? Never! Hand to God and cross my heart, the owner lives on the twenty-second floor of the Lincoln Towers. He's an actor in a soap. Came home after work and threw open the window to get some air. Thought a screen was there, but the super had taken the screens down for the winter. The dumb cat just dove right out. If the cat lives, the guy's gonna give me an affidavit saying the apartment's on the twenty-second floor. Then the loot's mine, all mine!"

"Remember, Kenny, you don't have to catheterize him," I laughed.

"I know. He peed on the way down from fright. Hope no one was standing under him. Talk about your acid rain," he snickered.

"What pool're you talking about? I didn't know there was any pool." Hartley was offended.

"Maybe you were absent that day," Kate shouted over her cat's yowl.

"It's the High-Rise Cat Pool," I explained. "Anytime one of us gets a cat that's jumped from a window—"

"Or been pushed," Kenny interjected.

"Yeah, or thrown," I went on, "we put a buck in the pool, and at Christmas, the one who treated the cat that fell from the highest floor and lived—wins."

"I think that's sick!" Hartley sneered. "We're supposed to be saving animals' lives, not betting on whether they're gonna die."

"Oh, Hartley, give me a break." Kenny was exasperated. "We're not betting on whether they're gonna die. We're betting on how far they've fallen and whether they're gonna live. Don't be an asshole all your life. Anyway, when you go back to Petula Falls, or wherever it is you're from, you won't have to worry about high-rise cats. There probably isn't a building over two stories in the whole town."

"It's Pebula Falls, with a *B*," Hartley corrected him. "And there aren't any buildings over *four* stories, and there aren't any smart asses like you either, thank God. Just plain simple people who have their values straight."

"Good. Perfect place for you. You can go back and play James Herriot in the Yorkshire Dales. I just pity the poor animals you have to treat on your own!" Kenny was angry now, and wimpy Hartley was no match for him.

"OK, guys, enough!" I cut in. "There's a waiting room out front filled with animals and people, and we're all back here jawing. Now let's get moving. Hartley, you get out there and call your next case. I'll finish up and take the Lhasa to X-ray. Go on, move it!"

I didn't like Jim Hartley any more than Gilbert did. He was a self-righteous whiner, who unfortunately wasn't very good at his chosen profession. He was no better with animals than he was with people. Some vets, even if they aren't medical whizbangs, have what I like to call "good hands," the ability to communicate to animals through manner and touch an immediate sense of trust. Many animals are terrified by visits to the vet. If they're in pain or suffer trauma, the terror is compounded and, unless they're unconscious when they're brought in, their confidence must be won. You have to talk to them, soothe them. You can't stride into a treatment room and whisk a dog off the floor and onto the table without so much as a "how do." Like humans, animals appreciate a reassuring bedside manner. Hartley just didn't have it. In his three months at the hospital, he'd been bitten four times, a record unequaled as far as I know. Animals do have a sixth sense; I think the dogs were trying to tell us something.

I wondered how Jim Hartley had managed to get a prized place as an intern at the AMC and why he wanted to be a vet in the first place. It's not a profession one just falls into. There's too much work and too many years of training involved. For most of us, it's the culmination of a lifelong love for animals and the desire to work with them and help them. For some, it's a fairly respectable way to make a decent living. But a few see dealing with animals as a means of avoiding people, though the fallacy in that soon becomes apparent, particularly in urban veterinary practice where people and their animals are often inseparable. To treat one you must relate to the other. It seemed Hartley was unable to do either.

"I'm sorry, Steve. Didn't mean to get so ticked off. That guy is such a jackass, he makes my blood boil." Kenny went back to cleaning a laceration on his high-rise victim.

"He's just overwhelmed by it all. Maybe he'll straighten out," I offered lamely, knowing it would never happen.

"What makes you so charitable all of a sudden?" Kate flared. "You're the one ends up doing his work for him."

"Like my grandmother used to say, 'He can't help himself, poor soul.' He's a schlepper, a misfit. I kind of feel sorry for him," I shrugged.

I lifted Harry back onto the rolling stretcher. Susan had cleaned the blood off his face and ears. Now that I was certain he was stable, we would take him to X-ray. I looked over at Kenny again. "How's your fifty-buck cat doing?"

"In the pink, in the pink!" He made a circle with his thumb and forefinger.

"Well, if you have any problem, call me. Then we can split the fifty," I laughed.

"Not a chance. This little bugger's gonna make it. He has to—he's the price of the booze for my Christmas party."

"I'll drink to that!" Kate had finished unblocking her cat's urethra. He had finally stopped yowling and now was slung over her shoulder like a baby she was about to burp. "Call *me*. I'll *contribute* my half!"

Susan and I rolled Harry into radiology. We transferred him to the X-ray table, careful not to dislodge the IV catheter.

"Chest, abdomen and head," I instructed Ito, the technician.

Five minutes later, after Harry had been comfortably arranged in an ICU cage with heat lamps, I was back out front talking with his owner. She really was a knockout. About that, Hartley was right. Tall, maybe five feet eight, and slender as a model, she moved with an athletic grace. Her clothes were casual, but elegant. Well-cut black trousers topped by a soft, black silk shirt open at the throat, and at her waist, a black belt with a large, smooth silver buckle. The bloodied jacket she still clutched was a gray and black herringbone tweed.

"Do you really think he'll be all right? If anything happens to that dog, I'll never forgive myself." The concern showed in her face.

"He's looking pretty good at this point, so I'd be encouraged. The X rays are clear, no broken bones. Although as I explained, with head trauma, it's a question of watching the neurologic function over a period of time."

"Is there any possibility of brain damage?" Her hazel eyes darkened.

"I'd hope not. But I'll keep a close watch on him and see how he responds tonight. Try not to worry; I think he'll pull through this just fine. He's young, and aside from the accident, he seems very sound. You can call me at any time, if you're worried, and if you like, I'll call you later on this evening." I was trying to allay her fears, but I wasn't above promoting any extended relationship that might result from Harry's misfortune.

"You're very kind, Doctor—umm—Kritsick." She looked at the plastic nameplate on my lab-coat pocket. "I've never had occasion to come here before, and I didn't quite know what kind of treatment we'd get."

"Only the best. Don't worry, we'll get Harry in shape. I'm certain of it."

"Poor darling. It really is my own damned, dumb fault. We've been in California, and I left him with my mother for a week. She lives in Brooklyn Heights and hasn't been too well, so she didn't exercise him. I got back yesterday, and when I picked him up tonight, he was so excited and pleased to see me, I took him out for a run. My mother lives on a very quiet street. There's usually no traffic, and besides, Harry always stays on the sidewalk. I let him off the lead. Yes, I know I shouldn't have done it," she said quickly, afraid I might chastise her. "He just took off at fifty miles an hour, darted between two parked cars with me screaming after him. Then this car came barreling down the street. It was dark, the driver didn't see him—" she paused, her eyes filling with tears as she relived the moment. Her voice caught when she spoke again. "It was just awful. You know, if you love someone very much, sometimes you have those dreadful flashes of something terrible happening to them. I adore Harry. He's a great little dog, and I have those flashes about him. Suddenly, there it was, really happening. My heart truly stopped. I suppose that's the price you have to pay for caring, whether it's for a child, a man, or a dog."

"Isn't it worth it when you get so much in return?" I asked.

"I'm not questioning that for a minute. It's just an observation, Doctor. Loving Harry is wonderfully easy. He accepts me just as I am and wants no changes or compromises, as far as I know."

"A very wise dog Harry is, with exceptionally good taste. Knew it the minute I laid eyes on him."

Her tears stopped, and she smiled. But whatever points I'd scored as kindly, understanding Dr. Kritsick would soon be erased by the crassness of what I now had to bring up—money. Usually, I have no problem talking about it. The cost of an animal's stay in this hospital is a fact of life that simply must be dealt with. But it would have been nice not to have to discuss it with Andrea Walker. After all, we'd been talking about big stuff, life and death and love. If this were an old movie, Harry would just be taken care of, never a fee involved. Beautiful girls never discussed money with their kindly vets. It was too petty.

"Now, the estimate for Harry's treatment, including the X rays and his overnight stay, is about $300," I began the litany. "You can pay half of it now and the rest when Harry's released." It sounded as if I were talking about time payments on a new dishwasher, lines Jimmy Stewart never would've uttered to Katharine Hepburn. "When the medical service checks him tomorrow morning, they'll see if any additional treatment is needed, and the bill will be adjusted accordingly. OK?"

"Fine, Doctor," she nodded. "I don't care what it costs. Whatever it is, it's worth it!"

Good, that was done. Now back to kindly Dr. Kritsick, circumventing hospital routine for gorgeous Andrea Walker. "If there's anything dire, the medical service will call you—or better still, I'll talk with them and call you myself. You'd better give me a phone number where you can be reached at all times." Before I was even out of vet school, I learned the best way to a girl's heart was often through her dog. It might still be true.

She pulled a business card out of a small, finely made leather case and handed it to me.

Walker & Walker
Public Relations
439 East 57th Street
New York, N.Y. 10022
(212) 756-4878

"Who's the other Walker?" I asked, hoping it was her brother, at worst.

"That's my husband, Brian. He's still in Los Angeles. He's as nutty about Harry as I am. Thank goodness I can tell him everything's all right."

Thank goodness, indeed! Oh well, scratch one for kindly Dr.

Kritsick. The very least she might've done was correct me when I called her *Miss* Walker.

"DOCTOR KRITSICK TO THE PREP ROOM, EMERGENCY! DOCTOR KRITSICK, PREP ROOM PUL-EAZE!" The call resounded through the reception area. I quickly filled out Harry's treatment record and escorted *Mrs.* Walker to the cashier.

"Thank you again, Doctor Kritsick. I'm going to tell all my friends how super you are."

"My pleasure," I assured her and ran back down the corridor to the prep room.

Kenny's fifty-dollar cat had gone sour. The trauma of the fall had caused an accumulation of air in the chest cavity, what we call a pneumothorax. The free air was interfering with the lungs' ability to expand, and now the cat could barely breathe. That he was alive at all was a miracle. After all, twenty-two stories is an enormous distance. But to keep him alive, we would have to tap his chest and get the air out.

"I was hoping he'd make it on his own without the tap. I've never done one before, Steve." For the first time, Kenny seemed unsure of himself.

"That was wishful thinking, pal. But there's nothing to it. After this guy, you'll be an expert. Let's take a look at the rads."

Kenny slapped the X rays on the prep-room light panel. I could see from the dark shadows that the accumulation of air was much greater on the left side, under the fractured ribs, than on the right. If we could relieve the pressure there, the lungs would function properly again. Between his labored breaths, the cat moaned pathetically. The broken ribs were evidently causing pain, but we couldn't sedate him. That would only depress his system further. We would just have to work as quickly as possible.

While Kenny held the cat down on its right side, I shaved the hair on its left chest with electric clippers and swabbed the area with Betadine scrub and then alcohol. I attached a 22-gauge hypodermic needle about an inch and a half long to a slender piece of extension tubing with a three-way stopcock valve at the end.

Then I hooked a large 35-cc syringe to the valve.

"OK, Kenny, let's change places." I handed him the needle and the syringe and I held the cat. Kenny's curly, yellow hair had gone wild and was falling over his eyes, already wide with apprehension.

"Come on, you can do it," I urged him on. "If we don't work fast, this cat's a goner and so's your party. Now, you're gonna go in between two ribs, I think the sixth and seventh might be best. Try and get the needle in at an angle, so you don't puncture a lung or hit the heart."

"Bite your tongue," Kenny said, concentrating so hard, the perspiration ran in little rivulets down his nose and the side of his head. The cat howled when he inserted the needle between the two ribs. "Sorry, feller. It'll only hurt for a second, hang in there with me—just another instant—there! It's in! Now what?"

"Good. Now open the stopcock valve and pull back on the plunger. If you've hit air, it'll come back easily. If you haven't, you'll know it."

Kenny struggled with the syringe plunger. "Shit! I can't get it back. Damn!"

Somehow, in the great mass of air in the cat's chest, Kenny had found a vacuum. He would have to try again. I suggested tapping between the eighth and ninth ribs, staying well away from the fractured ones. "Close the valve when you withdraw the needle and open it again as soon as the needle is back in," I told him.

The cat, though in no shape to talk back, emitted a scream of protest when Kenny pushed the needle through the chest wall and between its ribs for the second time. He opened the valve and slowly pulled back on the plunger. As he did, a satisfied smile played across his face. "It's coming, by God, it's coming! This is terrific, Steve. It's like striking oil—easy when you know where to look."

His confidence restored, Kenny whistled while he repeated the process several times, eventually drawing almost 300 cc of air from the cat's chest. "There you go little Pyewacket, baby mine," he crooned, "You're gonna be all better in no time, and nice Doctor Gilbert is gonna have his party after all."

"Pyewacket? That his name? What kind of name is that for a cat?"

"It's from some play. His owner's an actor."

"Oh yeah, right. In a soap."

"He plays a doctor, I think."

"Why are they always doctors? Why can't anyone ever be a vet?"

"Why Doctor Kritsick, do I detect a note of yearning in your voice? Maybe some TV producer is in the waiting room now as we speak, and we'll save his old dog Rover. Money cannot possibly repay us, so in our honor he'll produce a new television series, *Young Dr. Kritsick and His Faithful Sidekick, Younger Doctor Gilbert, Saviours of Suicidal Cats and Very Old Dogs.* What d'ya think? Will it play in Pebula Falls?"

"What do they know in Pebula Falls from suicidal cats? Nevertheless, this guy seems to be coming around. His breathing's much better. His color's good. I venture to say, he's gonna live. Doctor Gilbert, I think we've done it!"

"By George, you're right, Doctor Kritsick. I think we have!"

Kenny carefully lifted Pyewacket, the limp, calico wonder cat, from the treatment table and put him on the rolling stretcher. He would be taken to ICU and settled in a cage, where he'd be kept warm with heat lamps and monitored throughout the night. Now that his breathing was relatively normal, only rest, supportive care and time would heal the broken pelvis and the fractured ribs. No surgery would be necessary. Pyewacket was an extraordinarily lucky cat. He survived a fall that by all rights should've splattered him on the pavement like a batch of scrambled eggs. But then, I think that every time I see a high-rise victim who lives—and in warm weather I see at least four or five a week. High-rise syndrome is a fact of feline life in New York, and surviving its consequences may be just another indication that Darwin's theory of adaptation is still at work. On the other hand, we don't know which cats fall accidentally and which ones jump because they simply can't take it anymore.

"Oh, by the way, Gilbert—" I caught him just as he was half-way out the prep room door. "You owe me twenty-five bucks!"

"Well, Jesus, Steve, aren't you gonna contribute it?"

"Contribute it? What am I, a philanthropist?"

"You want the Christmas party, don't you?"

I smiled. "I'll take it under advisement."

Chapter 10

That first summer in New York, August was even hotter and more uncomfortable than July. After five days of temperatures well over 90°, waves of heat rose from the pavement, and the heels of my shoes squished in the melting asphalt when I stepped off the curb at Columbus Circle to cross the street and enter Central Park. What we needed was rain. Thunderstorms had been predicted, and the sky had darkened several times with the promise of a cloudburst, only to brighten again as the heavy clouds passed over without releasing so much as a cooling drop.

It was Saturday, and like so many other New Yorkers trapped in the city without a car and unwilling to struggle to the beach on a crowded subway or bus, I would try to claim a patch of grass for myself at the side of Central Park's lake. At least it was water, and looking at water, even if it was polluted, was certainly better than sweltering in my apartment. I had seen every movie in town but one, and that air-conditioned delight I was saving for tonight.

As I darted across the street against the light, narrowly beating the cars rushing down Central Park South toward the circle, I noticed a large crowd gathered around an open Victoria carriage in front of the park's entrance. The white ASPCA horse ambulance was parked directly behind it, and when I got closer, I saw why. The horse that had been pulling the Victoria had literally dropped in its traces and now lay sweating on the hot pavement. Its eyes, frightened and wide, rolled back so the whites showed as it tried in vain to lift its head. A fat, sweaty man I assumed to be its owner stood over it, his hands jammed in the pockets of his dirty khaki pants, his short-sleeved Hawaiian shirt open over a stained white undershirt barely covering his hairy belly. On his head was a battered black silk opera hat of about the same vintage as the carriage.

"Why dontchya give the poor horse some water, ya creep?" a woman onlooker yelled at him, and there was a chorus of agreement from the crowd.

"I did! Whadya want from me? I did!" The man screamed back.

"This horse shouldn't've been on the street in the first place. Not on a day like this. We've warned you before." I recognized Walter Schroeder, the cruelty agent from the A. He spoke sharply to the man and then knelt by the prostrate horse. I elbowed my way through the group and crouched next to him.

"Doctor Kritsick, what're you doing here?" Walter was startled to see me.

"I just happened to be passing and saw the crowd and your truck. But it doesn't look like I can be much help now."

"No," Walter sighed. "Once they're down like this, they're finished. If he doesn't go by himself in the next few minutes, I'll have to put him out of his misery." He fingered the holstered .38 revolver at his side. "I have to get this guy to sign the release first."

As Walter Schroeder stood up, the horse, an old black gelding, tried again to lift its head. Then it shuddered and was suddenly still, the heavy lather from its coat forming small puddles beneath it. There would be no need now for Walter to use the gun, nor for the owner to sign the consent release.

The horse-drawn hansom cabs and Victorias that line the broad avenues bordering Central Park, waiting to carry tourists or, occasionally, celebrating New Yorkers on nostalgic jaunts through the park, are one of the city's more romantic attractions. But the picturesqueness of the rigs from another, simpler time, often festooned as they are with colorful garlands of flowers, masks a problem that's been of deep concern to the ASPCA, the Humane Society and animal lovers in general for many years— the brazen abuse of those hundred or so horses by their owners and drivers.

The conditions under which the carriage horses live and work, with few exceptions, are deplorable. The stables are, for the most part, old, rundown and dirty. They're cold and drafty in winter and inhumanely hot in summer.

At that time, the horses could be forced to work no matter what the weather, and it wouldn't be until 1981 that a law was finally passed requiring they be moved to a shady area and sponged down when the outside temperature rose above 90°, and that they be taken off the streets altogether if it remained above 90° for more than three days. It's a statute that's made the horses' lot only slightly better, since it's often disregarded by owners anxious to make yet another fare. That summer, there was no law on the books other than the state's omnibus Cruelty to Animals Act, and under its provisions, Walter Schroeder had no provable grounds to give the owner of the fallen horse a summons for unusual abuse.

"He just worked him till he dropped." Walter shook his head in disgust. "He don't give a damn. He'll just take himself upstate and pick up another at auction for practically nothing. Then he'll treat that one the same way. In this weather, those horses should be off the streets. But there's nothing I can do. This time, I can't even haul him into court for a violation."

Walter Schroeder was the Chief Cruelty Agent at the ASPCA. He and ten other uniformed agents were responsible for the investigation and prosecution of all animal cruelty and abuse complaints in New York's five boroughs, an almost impossible task, considering the size of the city's animal population. When the weather was hot, Walter's job became even more difficult, especially with the carriage horses.

When it's extremely hot and humid, horses must be cooled down frequently. Unlike dogs, they sweat profusely when they're overheated. But also unlike dogs, they have no basic instinct to lie down and rest when they're exhausted. They must depend upon their human caretakers to see to it that they're sponged off in a cool place. Otherwise, at their owner's bidding, they just keep working. If a horse is pushed on a very hot day, the combination of work load and unusually warm environment can raise the animal's body temperature to over 108°, bringing about an imbalance in the electrolytes in the horse's system and, eventually, heat prostration. Once that happens, it's almost always irreversible, since there's no practical means of swiftly administering the many liters of fluid necessary to cool off a horse weighing a thousand pounds or better. The animal goes down, immediately becomes comatose and quickly dies. Such was the case with the black gelding.

The crowd had grown larger. Now that the horse was dead, morbid curiosity dictated the group remain standing in the hot sun gaping at the corpse until it was removed by the Sanitation Department truck summoned by Walter Schroeder's assistant. A dead horse in the streets of New York was an unusual event, an odd distraction from the discomfort of the unbearable heat that August afternoon. I noticed one man raise his little boy up on his shoulders so the child would have a better view. I wondered if it would have any impact on the boy in years to come, or if he would process it as simply another sidewalk curiosity, just as his father had done.

There was no need for me to hang around longer. I could be of no help to Walter Schroeder. I left him filling out his ASPCA forms and walked into the park, hoping to erase the image of the prostrate black horse as quickly as possible.

I've always had a very special feeling about horses. Powerful, gentle, intelligent and sometimes incredibly beautiful, they're capable of establishing unique relationships with human beings. That they could be deliberately abused and mistreated in full view of passersby, with the authorities doing little or nothing to stop it, made me furious.

Why, I wondered, couldn't the city build and supervise a stable for carriage and riding horses right here in Central Park? Certainly there was room for one. The money could be privately raised from the many horse lovers in the area, so it wouldn't cost the taxpayers a cent. What a terrific idea!

By the time I had picked my way between and through the hordes of sunbathers and picnickers and found my own spot under a gnarled maple at the side of the lake, I had completely constructed the new stable in my mind. Heated in winter and air-conditioned in summer, it would be every horse's delight. I, of course, would be the veterinarian in charge.

I watched the armada of rental rowboats being oared every which way across and around the lake. Some were made of worn, battered wood, others of graffiti-scarred metal. Their occupants, young and old and of all colors, sought relief from the incessant heat by shipping oars and trailing their hands or dunking their feet in the murky water. A few boys, heedless of the consequences to their future health, amidst much laughing and shouting, found some excuse to fall or be pushed overboard.

About fifteen yards from my shore, two boats, each containing at least six Hispanic kids, had hitched up. Their enormous portable radios tuned to the same station, playing at full volume, treated the other boaters to a free, if unsolicited, rock concert.

From where I sat I had a perfect view of the West Side skyline and the elegant apartment houses that line Central Park West—the Dakota, the Beresford, the Majestic, the El Dorado. The landscaped terraces of their luxurious penthouses looked down on the lake's Saturday sailors, though I was certain the people who lived in those expensive apartments were probably somewhere else—the Hamptons, Nantucket, or maybe even Europe. No one who had a choice would ever spend a hot August weekend in the steaming city.

I leaned back against the tree and closed my eyes, letting the sounds of music and laughter from the lake wash away the awful memory of what had taken place on the hot pavement outside the park.

Soon horses began to race through my mind. Beautiful, free, unbridled horses, the ones I had tended for three years as a vet student at Michigan State University. With them came the clear remembrance of the odd old recluse, Del Bennett.

I was paid $25 a week to feed and water a small herd of twenty-four mares donated to the university for breeding research. The project involved trying to synchronize the mares' heat cycles by using a small pony we called Horny as a tease. The idea behind this was, if all the mares in a stable came into season at once, it would expedite the breeding process. Whether a stallion or artificial insemination was used, you could just go down the line and bang, bang, bang! When I graduated from vet school, the research was still going on, and as far as I know, the plan has yet to succeed.

The horses were kept about two miles away from the Michigan State campus on a farm given to the university by a local benefactor, Del Bennett, Sr., with the proviso that his only son, Del, Jr., could live in the small shack on the property until he died.

Del, Jr., was a spooky legend around the vet school. We all knew about him; he was "mental." About sixty-five, he never washed or changed his clothes, and he lived by himself in his dirty, newspaper-cluttered shack without electricity or running water, speaking to no one. During the warm weather, he grew most of his food in a tiny garden next to the horse barn. The rest was brought to him by a county social worker who also came by every year before winter set in to take Del off to the state hospital where he would remain until spring. When Del returned to the farm each May, washed, shaved and wearing a new set of clean denims, we knew the harsh Michigan winter was over. Summer and Del Bennett, Jr., always arrived at the same time.

That first semester on the job, I was so caught up with the horses, I forgot completely about Del. Some of them were extraordinarily beautiful thoroughbreds that could no longer be used for racing, and, to me, just to watch them run free in the field was payment enough for tending them. One in particular became my special horse. She was a roan named Torrent, who had been relegated to the research project when an almost imperceptible lameness prevented her from making the quick stops and turns necessary for a top polo pony. The game's loss was my gain. I set about teaching myself to ride her bareback. And though, at first, every time I tried to mount her she tossed me with arrogant pleasure, after a few weeks of daily persistence, she must've realized I wouldn't give up, and we finally became good friends. Using nothing more than a rope for a bridle, I rode her every afternoon. In the beginning, we stayed in the paddock. But then as I became more secure, we ventured out into the broad, rolling meadows and hills behind the farm. She liked the exercise, and I loved the wondrous sense of freedom that came with cantering this high-spirited animal. Without a saddle, it was me and her and nothing between us.

One warm afternoon in early June after Torrent and I had been out for a particularly long ride, I brought her back to the paddock to water her and sponge her down. The drinking trough was an old bathtub that had to be filled by pumping water by hand from a well outside the paddock fence. A Rube Goldberg spoutlike contraption was connected to the pump and spilled water through the fence into the tub. If I pumped hard, it usually took about ten minutes to fill it.

Perspiration ran down my face and chest from the exertion necessary to push up and down on the handle of the ancient, rusty pump. The tub was almost filled, when I heard a soft rustling in the tall grass behind me. I looked over my shoulder and saw nothing. Maybe it was a rabbit, or the wind, or my imagination. I went back to the pump. Torrent was already drinking from the makeshift trough and she'd been joined by some of the other horses. Then I heard it again, a distinct sound of movement in the high grass, like an animal or maybe— I turned quickly, and as I did, I saw him rise from the green underbrush like a ghostly apparition, so startling me that I fell back against the fence and almost through it into the bathtub.

He was tall and sickly thin. His grimy denim pants and shirt, at least a size too big, emphasized his spare frame. His face was covered with field dust and wisps of straggly grayish brown beard that matched the long, matted hair on his head. His dark eyes were hollows so deep it was difficult to read their expression. His cheeks, gray from the dust, were sunken, and his lips were folded in as if there were no teeth to support them.

He stood still for a moment, then shambled toward me with his hand outstretched, a toothless grin splitting his face. I knew this had to be Del Bennett. I shouldn't have been frightened of him; he was a helpless old man. But I was. Maybe it was the countless stories I'd heard about crazy Del. I pushed farther back against the fence, wondering how long, for how many days he had lain in the grass and silently watched me, or peered at me from the dirt-encrusted, cracked windows of the shack.

He came closer. Now I could smell him, an acrid sour smell, strong and unpleasant. Not like the clean, sweet manure smell of the horses, I loved that. Without a word, he took my hand in his. It was rough and leathery. He pulled me away from the pump, gesturing with his head toward the shack about fifty feet down the hill.

"What do you want me to do?" I asked him. But he didn't answer. I didn't know if he could speak. After the initial shock, I was no longer afraid, and I let him lead me through the slatted door that swung half open on one rusty hinge and into the dilapidated structure. In the four months I had worked at the farm, I had never been inside the shack. If nothing else, I was curious.

The windows were so filthy they allowed little light into the small room, and it took a few seconds for my eyes to adjust to the semidarkness. When they did, I saw stacks of newspapers piled in sagging heaps covering almost every inch of floor space, except for one corner, in which there was a cot with no sheet on the torn mattress, just a soiled army blanket folded over the metal rail at its foot. There was no other furniture in the room. No table, no chair, and certainly there wasn't a kitchen or bath. Del had no use for them. He neither cooked nor washed, and I assumed he used the outdoors for a toilet, though the stench in the room was so overpowering, I had second thoughts about that.

Now that I had seen the shack from the inside, I wanted to get out as quickly as possible. But the old man had moved aside a five-foot pile of newspapers and was pointing strenuously to an old-fashioned wooden icebox they had hidden. He evidently wanted me to help him move it outside.

I pushed some of the newspapers away to make a path to the door, took a deep breath, put my shoulder to the icebox and shoved it across the planked floor and out onto the rickety porch. Del Bennett nodded his head vigorously with approval and once again flashed his toothless smile. He was obviously elated by my success, though I couldn't imagine what he planned to do with the old box. But for some secret reason I'd never know, it was important to him, and that would have to suffice.

"Is there anything else you'd like me to do?" I asked him. He motioned me to wait on the porch, and he disappeared into the darkness of the shack. In a few moments he returned carrying a heavy, tarnished brass medallion about two inches in diameter. He handed it to me, indicating it was mine to keep.

I held it up in the bright sunlight and made out blackened letters that read Souvenir of the World's Fair—New York 1939. Above the letters were the symbols of the fair, the trylon and perisphere. I wondered how he had gotten it. Perhaps his father had visited the fair and brought it home for him. Perhaps he'd just found it somewhere. In any event, from the look of the shack, it was probably one of his few possessions, and he'd given it to me as a thank-you.

That was the beginning of the odd relationship I was to have with Del, Jr., for the next several years. He never spoke to me. But every so often, after he'd seen I was finished caring for the horses, he'd make it known that he wanted me to help him carry something in or out of the shack. In return, he'd give me a present—anything from a potato or a carrot, to an old glass bottle. I had to accept it. That's the way things were between us.

Not too long ago, I heard that Del Bennett's shack had burned to the ground and he was killed in the fire. I still have the medallion he gave me. I've shined it up and I use it as a paperweight. Every time I look at it, I think of Del and my horses, especially Torrent. I had wanted to bring her back East with me when I finished vet school, but the impracticality of that scheme was readily apparent, even to me. I could barely afford to feed myself while I was interning at Angell, much less a horse.

I was suddenly aware that the tenor of the noise from the lake had changed. The rock music was still resounding loudly across the water, but the laughing had become angry shouts and screams. I looked up to see that the two other rowboats filled with teenage boys had collided with the music makers, and a full-scale naval battle was now underway. Three dark-haired girls in the first boats cheered on their boyfriends as they beat off the marauders with oars and beer cans. I had the feeling the fight was going to turn nasty, and I didn't want to witness it. I'd had enough ugliness for one day.

I left my shady spot under the tree and walked across the park toward 72nd Street, hoping not to see any more carriage horses working in the hot sun. Before I went to the movies tonight, I would write a letter to the Mayor's Office describing my plan for a stable in the park. Who could tell—someone might even read it.

Chapter 11

I would've sold my soul for a cold beer. Anything to zip up my flagging energy and get me through the next two hours. But the stream of patients at the Animal Medical Center was endless. There was no time to nip upstairs to the fourth-floor cafeteria and do battle with vending machines that were usually out of order. I made do with half an Oreo cookie someone had left unattended on the counter in the night pharmacy.

You'd have thought we were giving away free lottery tickets with every examination. If only there had been a good mini-series on television, we'd be seeing just the most serious cases. Then my head wouldn't be pounding and my legs wouldn't feel as if I'd just run the Boston Marathon.

I've always thought our waiting room was a much more accurate barometer of television fare than the Nielsen Ratings. When *Roots* or *The Holocaust* or *Shogun* were on, you could have shot off a cannon in that room and hit neither man nor beast. But here it was 10:30 P.M., and at least fifty people had forsaken *Quincy* and *Dynasty* for the thrills and chills of the Animal Medical Center.

I picked up the next clipboard with the patient's record attached, off the counter near the door. I had lucked out for a change. It was a collie who needed a simple booster shot. I would have him in and out in five minutes.

"Oh, thank God you're here, Steve!" Kate Gilchrist slid into the pharmacy at a run. She grabbed the clipboard from my hand and threw it back on the counter. "Don't call your next case; I need you desperately!" Her face was chalk white. She was as agitated as I'd ever seen her. "There's a python in Booth 6," she gasped.

"Yeah, so?" I knew what was coming.

"So I can't handle it," she said flatly. "I'll throw up!" She nervously fingered the stethoscope around her neck. "I thought I could. I wanted to—I wanted the challenge. And Hartley ducked it, so I took the case. But when the boy got the damned thing out of the carrier and it slithered around his neck and onto the table, I couldn't even look at it, much less touch it!" She shuddered, and her color went from white to a kind of green tinge. The crack in her voice was even more pronounced, "Please, Steve, would you look at it? Just this once—I'll owe you," she pleaded.

She was hard to resist, but I stood firm. "You already owe me for the iguana last month."

"I can't help it, Steve; they all give me the willies."

"I don't like them any better than you do. They give me the willies too," I grumped. "You guys have to learn how to deal with exotics. What're you gonna do in private practice, when I'm not there?"

"That's one of the reasons I'm specializing in cardiology," she laughed. "When was the last time you heard about open-heart surgery on a snake?" She had regained her sense of humor as well as her color. Kate was a terrific intern, and she rarely avoided difficult cases. I couldn't have her throwing up all over the exam table. It wouldn't be seemly at the Animal Medical Center.

"OK, I'll do it," I told her. "But only if you'll have dinner with me on Saturday night."

"You've got it!" She smiled with relief. I could have been Jack the Ripper, and she would have agreed. Anything not to handle the snake. She happily went off with my collie, and with great trepidation, I went to Booth 6.

If you want the truth, I can't bear snakes. Probably, I hate them even more than Kate does. I get goose bumps the minute I touch one. The phobia—and I guess that's what it is—began when I was interning at Angell.

I had been there only two weeks. Everything was still unfamiliar and a little forbidding—the way it is when you go from elementary school to high school and the desks are so big and you don't yet know your way to the chem lab or the boys' room. After all the years of fantasizing, I was finally wearing the greens of an Angell intern. I looked the part, but I still didn't feel I belonged. I was certain someone was going to tap me on the shoulder and say, "You—OUT!"

Though Angell Memorial Animal Hospital was not as large as the Animal Medical Center, it was overwhelming compared to the quiet rural atmosphere of vet school at Michigan State. When I arrived in 1974, the hospital was housed in the same old Victorian building I had visited eight years before with Emily Addison. But in the interim, the neighborhood had changed considerably, and though Angell was still thought to be the best animal hospital in the country, a large percentage of the clientele now came from the heavily ethnic population of the adjacent Roxbury line area. However, all of Boston regarded Angell with pride, and it was vigorously supported by a wide range of people from Back Bay and Beacon Hill to the South End, as well as by those who came to have their pets treated from the suburbs and as far away as Belgium and Hawaii.

But the color of the clients' skin, the language they spoke and their economic status was immaterial. Nothing I had learned at Michigan State prepared me for the catalog of urban veterinary experiences I encountered in those first weeks at Angell. I had learned how to make sick animals well. I knew little or nothing about the psychological quirks of the people who owned those animals—the obsessive attachments of city dwellers to their pets and the unspeakable abuses they sometimes inflicted on them.

A big-city animal hospital is a microcosm of the world outside, where love, hate and cruelty know no economic or social boundaries. The man who batters his dog often batters his wife and children. The woman who is kind to her animals is usually just as kind to the kids living down the street. There are exceptions, of course, and through the years I've become pretty adept at spotting them. But for the most part it's a rule that holds true.

Another rule is that people express themselves not only through their treatment of their pets but through their very choice of the animal. There are dog people, cat people, bird people and those I still find difficult to understand—reptile people. Who could love a snake, I wonder? Worship, perhaps. After all, snakes have been a part of almost every ancient mythology. Fear, maybe. There's always been the bad rap that first snake got in the Adam and Eve story, and many snakes do have poisonous venom, which is indeed lethal. But love? Never. At least that's what I thought until I ran into Charlie, an eight-foot boa constrictor, and his owner, Cecily Robertson, a Candy Bergen look-alike, who was working in anthropology at Harvard.

She entered my clinic booth carrying a beat up Louis Vuitton suitcase, circa 1935, and without so much as a hello, slung it up on the treatment table.

"He hasn't eaten in a month and now he has these terrible sores on his neck and back. I'm worried sick!" She snapped the tarnished brass locks on the case and opened the lid to reveal the biggest snake I had ever seen outside of a Tarzan movie.

Like most vet schools, Michigan State gave short shrift to exotic animals. Aside from dogs, cats and horses, most of our class time was spent on livestock. I was a big man with cows, pigs, goats, sheep and chickens. And though the odds on finding any of those in downtown Boston were even longer than on meeting a snake, I was certainly better equipped to deal with them. Luckily, I had recently thumbed through a book on reptiles and recognized the monster now coiled in front of me as a boa constrictor—a large boa constrictor. When the case was opened and the light hit it, the snake raised its head and hissed loudly. I jumped back involuntarily.

"I hope you're not afraid of him, Doctor. Charlie's really a dear when you get to know him."

"I'm sure he is," I told her, certain of the fact that I had no desire for any kind of personal relationship with Charlie—or any snake, for that matter. It occurred to me, then and there, that I didn't like snakes—not one bit. But somehow, I had to get this one out of its case and at least make a cursory examination. I was embarrassed. I couldn't acquit myself badly in front of Cecily Robertson. If a little odd, she was an extraordinarily beautiful girl. The kind who makes you catch your breath. She was fair and slender, and her hair, the blondest of blond, fell to her shoulders. She reminded me of those sirens who sit on rocks in Germany. Her eyes were blue purple, the color of an iris, and her features were perfectly sculpted. Like I said, she was a dead ringer for Candy Bergen. What, I wondered, was a goddess like this doing with a snake like that?

I pulled myself together, summoning all of the professional courage I could muster, and reached into the case to lift the snake out. In vet school, I had gotten into a cage with a wild she wolf with a broken leg. That was easier; at least she had four feet and fur. I could talk to her. But this! The snake undulated its head and hissed again. Cecily interceded (in my mind, I was already calling her Cecily).

"Here, let me help," she said kindly, and rubbed her hand along the snake's scaly back. "That's a good boy, Charlie. Come on out so the doctor can look at you. Come on, be a good boy," she coaxed. "Come on."

At her touch, the snake wriggled out of the case so that half of its body was on the table. I could see the abscesses she was talking about. They were large and filled with pussy matter. I remembered enough from that one course in exotic animals to put on a pair of disposable surgical gloves to make a closer examination. Sometimes the bacteria that attack reptiles are transferable to humans.

"How long has he had these?" I asked.

"Just a few days, as far as I can tell. I've been away at a seminar. They weren't there when I left."

"Hmmm," I said professionally. If I had had a beard, I would have tugged it. "They look pretty bad. Bacterial infection. We'll have to do some cultures before I can tell you exactly what it is. Have you handled him a lot?"

"Quite a bit."

"Then you may have to get an antibiotic shot yourself. Now, not eating doesn't mean anything. Snakes can go for weeks without food. If he's lost a lot of body weight, that would mean something. Has he?"

"Some, I think."

I made much of studying the abscesses further. "What kind of seminar were you at?"

"Primitive religion. I'm an anthropologist."

"At Harvard?" That would be convenient. I was beginning to find Charlie less ominous. I even felt some concern for his awful sores.

"No, in New York. I mean the seminar was in New York, but I'm at Harvard. I'm working on my Ph.D."

It was impossible not to be impressed. How could anyone so beautiful be brilliant as well? For her to have gotten all the marbles, someone somewhere must have been really shortchanged. She was older than I, about twenty-eight, maybe even thirty. Her clothes were as worn and beat up as the suitcase Charlie traveled in. You could see she didn't care about them. Not that it mattered. With her face, she could have marched about in a barrel and been considered a fashion trend setter.

I realized I was terribly self-conscious about being a mere intern. I wished I were on staff—maybe Chief of Internal Medicine, that would have wowed her. I even would have settled for being a resident—anything but a lowly intern. But the longer we stood there, the more certain I became that HALF-BAKED was written deeply across my forehead, like Hester Prynne's scarlet A. Thank God, I was able to remember enough about snakes not to have made a complete idiot of myself.

Charlie lay on the table, absolutely still. He didn't wriggle, he didn't writhe. I wasn't positive what a healthy snake should look like, but one thing was sure, this one wasn't in the pink.

When I explained that we would keep him in the hospital for a few days so that the abscesses could be cleaned out and a culture made to determine their cause, her blue-purple eyes filled with tears. "You be careful with him," she warned. "I don't want anything done that will cause him pain."

"Of course not. We're here to help, not to hurt," I stammered self-righteously.

"Yeah, I know. I'm an anthropologist and my husband's a resident at Mass. General. We're all there to help until something really interesting comes along, and then maybe it's time to experiment. But not with Charlie! You just remember that!" She was sharp and very abrupt.

"We'll take very good care of him," I promised, my fantasy about her completely blown. First a snake, then a husband, and he was a resident, yet. It was as if she had been sent to cut me down to size in case I had gotten too full of myself. Only in this instance, I was already so nervous and insecure that was hardly necessary. Since she'd walked into the room, I felt I had shrunk at least four inches.

She must have noticed the pain my diminished stature caused. "I'm sorry," she said quietly. "I didn't mean to be so harsh. It's just that I'm terribly fond of Charlie. That may be difficult for you to understand; it is for everybody. After all, he's a snake. My husband won't go near him."

"No, no," I interrupted, "I understand completely. It's easy to get attached to living things, any living thing—even a snake." I'd said the wrong thing, but she paid no attention.

"I've had him for two years and I know his moods. He has a wonderful disposition." She patted the limp snake lovingly. "And I know now something's very wrong with him. A friend of mine down the street at Harvard Med said you people were the only ones who could treat Charlie properly."

"We'll do our best," I assured her.

She helped me coil the snake back in the case. I closed the lid and firmly snapped the locks, promising to call her as soon as a diagnosis had been made. As she turned to leave, I stopped her. I could contain myself no longer. I had to know. "What made you get Charlie in the first place?" I asked.

She threw her head back and laughed so that I actually heard the ha-ha. "Everyone wants to know that. It's really very simple. Nothing strange or mystical about it. My field is primitive religion, as I told you. Snakes, snake gods and snake worship play such an enormous role in so many nonliterate and ancient cultures, I thought it would be a good idea to get to know one first hand. So I got Charlie." She brushed her long hair back with her hand and leaned against the doorjamb. "I had no idea I'd get so attached to him. But I did. So much so that I'm doing my thesis on snakes and religion. He was the inspiration. He's real important to me and he's a love. So you will take good care of him for me, won't you, Doctor?" Her eyes traveled to the closed suitcase. She smiled and looked so ravishing, I'd have done anything for her and her snake, husband notwithstanding.

At Angell, when you admitted an animal, its case became your personal responsibility. With the help of your staff supervisor, you diagnosed the illness and treated it until the animal was well enough to go home. Staff specialists might be called upon for surgery or consultation, but the animal always remained in your care. The procedure at the Animal Medical Center is quite different. Though I may admit a patient at night and treat it initially, it's then turned over to the medical service the next day, and they follow the case through until the animal is released. Five or six different people can handle any one case. I've always thought this lack of continuity was confusing to the client and not half so instructive for the interns. There's something about the burden of responsibility that makes you really pay attention.

Charlie, then, was completely my responsibility. After Cecily Robertson left, I took him to the Exotics Ward, which was on the third floor, away from the other animals. The ward was maintained at a constant temperature of 85° F. and 60 percent humidity. The lights were automatically turned on and off every twelve hours, providing an ideal environment for birds, amphibians, chelonians and reptiles.

Then I called in Dr. Jerry Hanfer, the staff person most familiar with exotics. He agreed with my tentative diagnosis of a bacterial infection, and after anesthetizing the snake with halothane, helped me to clean out the abscesses with a solution of hydrogen peroxide. Hanfer had been at Angell for over fifteen years and was considered the leading reptilian expert in the country. He was almost as strange looking as some of his patients. Tall and spindly, he wore steel-rimmed glasses with lenses as thick as the bottoms of Coke bottles. The glasses always slid down his long, pinched nose. But he knew his stuff. He made it a point to be kind and helpful to inexperienced interns, to whom most exotic animals might as well have been creatures from the far side of the moon.

"I think you must consider the possibility of pseudomonas in those abscesses," he told me in a professorial tone. "If it's gone too far, it can be fatal, you know. So until we get the bacterial cultures, we'll go on the assumption that's what it is and treat accordingly with heavy doses of antibiotics."

I put Charlie in an isolation cage in a corner of the ward, and I looked in on him daily to clean the abscesses and continue his program of antibiotics. But after two days, he seemed no better. In fact, the abscesses were multiplying, and the ones we'd cleaned and debrided so carefully weren't improving. As Cecily had predicted, the more I worked with the snake, the better I liked him. Not that he was my new best friend, but I found I did have some feeling about his increasingly precarious condition.

The bacterial culture had confirmed Jerry Hanfer's suspicions of pseudomonas, a particularly virulent strain that was evidently not sensitive to the powerful antibiotics we were using. Now the snake seemed to be writhing in pain, and his ventral scales were elevated, a possible sign of meningitis, as well. If that were so, there was little I could do to help him, and when Dr. Hanfer looked at him, he agreed it would be most humane to put Charlie to sleep.

"When you call the owner for permission," he suggested, "why don't you ask if you can do a postmortem. It would be neat to find out what's really going on."

A postmortem! Jesus, I wasn't even certain I knew how to put the damned snake to sleep, and even though I was on more intimate terms with Charlie, the idea of carrying our relationship into the necropsy room was just ghastly. Alive he was bad enough. Dead? Yecck!

I reached Cecily Robertson late that afternoon. She was understandably upset when I told her about Charlie, but immediately agreed to have him euthanized, after I described the pain I thought he was in. The "post" was another story. That took a bit of fast talking. But she finally capitulated to my one-scientist-to-another approach, convinced that Charlie's death might help us find a cure for reptilian meningitis.

It was almost 9:30 when the last patient left the clinic. I wolfed a piece of cold pizza, left over from someone else's order, washed it down with a Coke from the machine and headed up to the Exotics Ward. This would be as good a time as any to dispatch Charlie.

The ward was dark and still when I opened the door. But the second I turned on the lights, using the manual switch, a piercing shriek shattered the quiet, almost knocking me out of my tennis shoes.

"Heee—re's Johnny! *Caw, caw.* Heee—re's Johnny!"

When my heart stopped pounding, I realized Ed McMahon had not made a surprise visit to the Exotics Ward at Angell Memorial Animal Hospital. The announcer was a voluble mynah, admitted that evening for a respiratory infection. He was quickly joined by the other avian residents in a chorus of cheeps and chirps, and suddenly, the room was alive with flapping wings and birdcalls. The light had made them think it was morning.

The mynah was perched in a cage directly opposite the snake's. He eyed me suspiciously as I pulled Charlie out and coiled him into the old suitcase Cecily had said we could keep. When I closed the lid and snapped the brass locks, the bird jumped from his perch, twining his talons on the cage door and screeched hysterically, "Heee—re's Johnny! *Caw, caw, caw.* Heee—re's Johnny!" He fluttered his wings and wildly flapped back and forth from door to perch. Maybe some sixth sense had alerted him to the snake's fate.

"Here's Johnny yourself!" I muttered. "Don't you know how to say anything else? If you think I want to do this, you're wrong. I don't! Those are just the breaks, bird. It could be you, you know."

I turned off the light, and silence immediately fell on the ward, as if someone had lifted the needle off a phonograph record.

Carrying the snake-filled suitcase and a book on reptilian anatomy I had picked up from the hospital library, I walked through the long, open brick colonnade to the necropsy room on the other side of the building. It was, in effect, Charlie's last mile.

Necropsy, small and white tiled, featured a long, stainless-steel operating table and a single, bright overhead operating light. Steel shelves lined the walls, displaying large glass jars filled with various bits and pieces of an animal's organs preserved in formaldehyde. On the scrubbed tile counter, the sterilized instruments for postmortems were neatly laid out.

The sickening smell of the formaldehyde permeated the room and invaded my nostrils, sending my sinuses into immediate hysterics. It was a chronic problem I had learned to deal with in vet school. Rather than have my nose run like an open faucet, leaking into the animal body cavity before me, I twirled two pieces of Kleenex and inserted one in each nostril, like a stopper. The white Kleenex ends hung down to my upper lip, giving me the look of an elephant walrus. It might look a bit odd, but it worked.

I donned a pair of disposable surgical gloves and removed Charlie from the case. Dr. Hanfer had told me there were two ways to euthanize a snake. It could be put in the freezer for several hours or its head could be chopped off. Neither alternative seemed particularly attractive. The idea of freezing anything to death was absolutely intolerable, and chopping off its head certainly wasn't much better. However, it was quicker and neater and, with anesthesia, relatively painless. No doubt, Charlie's final experience would be a lot nicer than Marie Antoinette's.

I found the large, shallow box with a transparent lid, used for anesthetizing reptiles, and coiled the big snake neatly in it. At this point, he was in dreadful condition and offered no resistance. I closed the lid and attached the hose from the halothane tank to a hole in the side of the box and turned on the gas. Within minutes, the snake was out cold. The effects of the halothane would last about fifteen minutes, giving me ample time to administer the coup de grace.

The room was dark except for the operating light, and when I lifted the inert snake out of the box, his long body cast eerie shadows on the wall. A rubberized apron covering my greens, I laid him out full length on the table and chose a large, machetelike knife from the instrument counter. After holding it over Charlie's neck and sighting down the big lethal blade, I raised the knife with both hands, high above my head. My shadow danced on the wall, as in a hideous horror movie come to life. Only this time, I was the mad scientist. Little Stevie Kritsick from Lexington, Mass., had become Dr. Cyclops. I desperately wished I weren't alone in the room. Why did I ever choose to do this damned thing by myself?

My heart pounding so hard I could hear it, I brought the knife back as far as I could and then, with all of my strength, down on the snake's neck. *THWACK!*

With one blow, the head was off. It fell with a thud on the floor and rolled under the table. When I stooped to pick it up, the jaws suddenly snapped open, revealing the snake's waggling, long, dark, forked tongue. I yelped and jumped at least a foot in the air, crashing back against the shelves and sending a jar containing a pair of cat kidneys flying across the room where it smashed on the wall, dripping kidneys and formaldehyde all over the floor.

I knew that kind of thing often happened with reptiles, as I've heard it does with humans. But never having been present at either kind of beheading, I just wasn't prepared for it. I caught my breath again, set the open-jawed head aside and, with a scalpel, prepared to skin the snake by making an incision at the top of the body.

As the scalpel cut through the leathery skin, I thought I felt the snake move. By then I was so spooked I was sure it was only imagination. But as I sliced further down the body, it not only moved, it wriggled. I stood back and watched as the headless body twisted, turned and finally slithered off the table, landing at my feet.

My skin crawled. My hands were as damp and cold as the decapitated snake. I was terrified. I wanted to run from the room, not giving a damn if the snake had meningitis, or chickenpox. If Jerry Hanfer was so bloody interested, why didn't *he* cut it up and find out. Indeed, he had offered, but like an idiot, I'd insisted on doing it myself. It would be a learning experience, a challenge. Some challenge. A few more like this one and I'd be ready for accounting school. A nice clean CPA playing with cold-blooded numbers, not chopping heads off cold-blooded snakes.

I had to see it through. Hanfer would be expecting a postmortem report in the morning. But more important, this would be the first major piece of work I had done since coming to Angell.

I lifted the snake off the floor, laid it carefully on the table and began to cut once again. This time, I held the body as firmly as I could. No damned snake was going to scare the liver and lights out of me. I was no longer calling him Charlie. When he lost his head, the slender thread of our relationship was cut with it. In my mind he became just *snake*.

With deft, quick strokes, my scalpel moved halfway down the length of the body. I was now the pure scientist, with no feeling or emotion about what I was cutting. Then it happened. Snake gave a mighty lurch and slid out of my hands, back onto the floor. All my resolve slid with it. My stomach turned, and the awful metallic taste of nausea was in my mouth. The sweet stench of the formaldehyde was unbearable. Leaving the snake where it was, I ripped the Kleenex from my nose and ran out the door into the empty hall, trembling. If this had been a movie I'd been watching, I would've covered my eyes for this scene.

It was after midnight when I returned to the necropsy room. I had spent the past hour sitting on the railing of the open colonnade, breathing fresh air and trying desperately to bring a sane perspective to what should have been a routine chore. Somewhere in the Old Testament, a plague of snakes is mentioned. I couldn't remember whether it was Job or the Jews who suffered them. It must have been the Jews. God had to know snakes are too much for one man to bear—even Job.

My snake lay on the floor where I had left it. I pushed it with my foot, first one end, then the other. There was no movement. Bravely, I lifted it onto the table, ready to try once more.

Now that the snake was finally still, like a dead snake should be, and I had my act somewhat together, I zipped along at a rather remarkable clip, fascinated by the strange anatomy, so different from a dog's or cat's or from any warm-blooded mammal's. The snake's heart is three-chambered, with two distinct auricles and a tapered ventricle. I found only one lung—the right, with just a tiny vestige of a left lung, and there was no diaphragm at

all. Snakes use their rib action to breathe. The anatomical varia-
tions were many, and I learned more each time I found and identified one.

I worked through the night, snipping and cutting sections of
this organ and that organ, carefully laying each piece in a small,
lidded plastic container with holes in the side, then dropping the
containers in jars of formaldehyde. There they would remain
until the histopathologist took them in the morning and made
cross sections of the tissue, hardening it with paraffin and then
slicing the sections paper thin with a special machine. Those sliv-
ers would be put on glass slides and looked at under the micro-
scope. I had taken special care to section the tissue at different
levels of the spinal cord. That's where the meningitis would
show, if it were present.

As it turned out, my initial stab-in-the-dark diagnosis wasn't
too far off base. Meningitis was indeed present in the spinal-cord
tissue. And, if that didn't kill the snake, the pseudomonas infection suggested by Jerry Hanfer, which had already formed lesions
in the lung, would have. I called Cecily Robertson to tell her the
results of the post, but mostly so she'd know Charlie hadn't been
put to sleep in vain. She thanked me profusely. "You're a dear for
calling," she told me. "If I ever have another animal, you're its
doctor!"

I could only hope and pray that whatever she got—it wouldn't
be a snake!

Back in Booth 6 of the Animal Medical Center, a pimply-faced
boy of about fifteen stood with the six-foot python draped casually around his shoulders.

"She's not eating, Doc, and she's got this sore on her back."
He indicated with his chin an area near the snake's head.

I felt the goose bumps rise on my arms. I hoped they didn't
show as I removed the python from the boy's shoulders and
placed it on the exam table. "How long since it's eaten?" I asked.

"About a week—and it's a *she*," he said sharply.

She lolled comfortably on the cold metal table. I noticed two
distinct bite marks in the middle of the snake's back.

"How long have you had her?"

"About a week. Got her in a pet store on Second Avenue. She's a real beauty, don't you think?"

I tried, without noticeable success, to whip up some aesthetic appreciation for my patient. It seemed to me, the boy, who was picking at the pimples on his face, and his pet were ideally matched. "It's a nice snake," I managed. "Didn't they tell you at the pet shop—snakes often don't eat for weeks, sometimes months? I wouldn't worry about its appetite."

"*Her* appetite," the boy insisted.

"Yeah, *her* appetite," I conceded. "Anyway, these sores on her back are bite marks, probably from some rodent she was being fed at the pet store. It was faster than she was."

While the boy stroked the snake's back, I swabbed the sores with iodine and treated them with an antiseptic ointment. "There, that should do it," I told him. "I'll give you some more ointment to apply at home. Use it twice a day, and if the sores don't clear up, call me." I gave him my card with the hospital phone number written on it.

The boy stopped picking his face and coiled the snake into the Campbell's soup carton he used as a carrier. He was halfway out the door when he turned and shook his head with a kind of sad resignation. "You know, Doc," he said, "she's really very nice when you get to know her."

Chapter 12

"DR. KRITSICK, RECEPTION! DR. KRITSICK TO RECEPTION, PUL-EAZE!"

Carmen headed me off before I got to the front of the desk and handed me a crumpled, dog-eared business card with most of the lettering obscured by dirt and stains. When I flattened it on the counter, I realized the card was mine. It was the one I had given out as a Senior Staff Clinician at the ASPCA Hospital, where I worked when I first came to New York. Carmen gestured with her head at a woman standing in the middle of the waiting room with her dog. "It's hers. She won't say nothin', just keeps pointing to the card. You know her, Dr. Kritsick?" Her eyebrows raised and her mouth puckered in disgust.

I looked at the woman, amazed to see both she and her dog were still among the living. There was no way I could've forgotten her.

"Yeah, I know her, Carmen. I'll take care of it," I told her.

"What about a record?" Carmen insisted. "She won't tell me her name, so I can't find no record."

"Don't worry about that," I assured her. "I'll take care of it." Not only was there no record, I knew there was no possibility the woman could pay for any treatment received. I would simply have to circumvent AMC red tape and handle it myself.

She was a bag lady. There were a lot of them in New York, but she was the only one I knew of who had a dog. She walked the streets (the Upper East Side was her beat), pushing a supermarket shopping cart filled with old newspapers, bottles, an ancient radio and two large shopping bags brimming with torn shoes and ragged clothes, treasures she had picked out of garbage cans along her route. Tied to the cart, which contained the sum total of all her worldly goods, was her dog, a medium-sized mixed breed, who walked at the same shuffling pace she did.

When I met her three years ago, it was winter. She and the dog were pressed against the bleak facade of the ASPCA building, seeking shelter from the icy wind and snow that whipped across York Avenue from the East River. The dog wore a makeshift coat fashioned from a piece of dirty red blanket. A rope tied around his middle kept it in place. The rest of the blanket was muffled around the woman's neck and shoulders, secured by a rusty safety pin.

If I looked closely, I could see she was dressed in layers, slight protection against the wet, biting cold. Beneath the tattered, buttonless army greatcoat, was a man's torn cardigan sweater and under that, a dress of sorts. Her blackened, scabby legs were bare, but for the rags twined around her shins and ankles, then down under her insteps in a sling effect to keep a pair of run-down carpet slippers on her feet. Like her legs, her hands and face were streaked with imbedded grime and soot, the result of endless days on the street and longer nights spent huddled in cold doorways. How she or any of the thousands like her survived was beyond me. They were human debris, ignored and overlooked much like dead leaves until they became too unsightly. Then they were swept away.

Coming from a relatively small town like Lexington, I was staggered by the numbers of men and women who lived in the streets of New York. At first, the sight of them crouched against buildings, or hunkered over sidewalk subway grates, garnering the meager benefit of the sightly warmer air coming through, so depressed me, I averted my eyes. They were like modern-day lepers placed in my path to test my charity. And in the beginning, I tried to meet the test by offering whatever money I had in my pocket to any and all of them. But I soon learned money wasn't always wanted. Sometimes, I was simply ignored, and on several occasions my well-meant gesture was met with a stream of invective and loud abuse.

Though the city provides shelters for the homeless, many are mentally unstable and incapable of finding these havens on their own. Others, for their own reasons, prefer the dangers of the streets to the crowded, institutionalized conditions of the city's "homes" and become well-known fixtures in whatever neighborhood they choose for themselves, living on handouts from local storekeepers and residents. New Yorkers aren't as cold and hard as the rest of the country would like to suppose. In fact, for the most part they're quite the opposite.

In the last six months I had been in New York, I had seen Lorraine (that was the only name she gave me) a couple of times on First or Second Avenue, noticing her especially because of the dog. I wondered what she fed him when finding food for herself must have been so difficult. I wondered where they slept—how they managed to get through each day and the even more treacherous nights. I wondered how she cared for the dog and if he ever had any shots. He was as dirty as she, but looked healthy enough. Once, I gave her two dollars, the only spare money I had in my pocket, which she accepted gratefully, flashing a gap-toothed smile.

That morning, walking with my head down against the bone-numbing chill, I hadn't seen her as I approached the door of the ASPCA. But she had spotted me. Perhaps she recognized me from our last encounter on the street. She tugged at the sleeve of my coat and pointed to the dog, who had a filthy, bloodstained rag wrapped around his leg.

"He's hurt, but I got no money," she rasped, her lips so cracked from the cold they barely moved when she spoke.

I doubted she knew I was a vet, but she did know this was an animal hospital and maybe I was someone who would help her. I motioned her inside and held the door while she pushed her cart into the lobby, the dog limping alongside.

With a slow, shambling gait, they negotiated the ramp that led to the second-floor clinic. When I offered to help her push the cart, she brusquely shoved me aside as if she were afraid I might make off with it and all the treasures it held.

Because of the early hour and the awful weather, the clinic

waiting room was empty. The rest of the hospital staff hadn't yet arrived. I led her into my treatment room and exchanged my wet overcoat for the white lab jacket I kept behind the door. I was glad no one else was there. I would be able to treat the dog as an emergency without having to worry about the usual fee requirement. Even at the ASPCA, where the majority of the clientele were ethnic poor, some payment was mandatory except in emergencies. Then we tried to help the animal as best we could, medicate it and send it on its way without hospitalization.

She stood by the table shivering in her wet clothes. Steam rose from the cold, soaked blanket on the dog's back.

"Why don't you take off your coat and his blanket," I suggested. "I'll get us some hot coffee from the machine."

When I returned bearing two paper cups filled with coffee, she took one from my hand and drank it greedily, oblivious to the liquid's scalding temperature. Her coat lay in a heap over the cart, and she tugged at the holey sleeves of the cardigan sweater, trying to cover her dirty arms. When I knelt next to her, to lift the dog onto the exam table, I was immediately aware of a strong, acrid odor surrounding her. It had probably been weeks, maybe even months, since she'd had a bath or washed.

The dog was part shepherd, part collie and maybe a little of something else impossible to identify. He seemed as wary of strangers as she was, and I spoke to him gently and reassuringly, before I lifted him onto the table. Once there, he knew instinctively I was going to help him. I felt no need for a muzzle or restraint. His coat was badly matted, and the injured leg was caked with blood. When I removed the soiled, wet rag, he whimpered softly, shifting his weight on the table.

"That's a good fella," I told him. "Try and hold still so I can see what you've done here." I sheared away some of the dirty hair with electric clippers and cleaned the wound with hydrogen peroxide. It was a nasty rip, about two inches long. It would need stitches.

"How'd this happen?" I asked the woman. She hadn't spoken a word since we entered the room.

"The box we was in last night, it had nails and I didn't know.

He must have got caught on 'em. I didn't know. I just seen all this blood." With the back of her hand, she swiped at a trickle of water that had come down her forehead from the wet wool army cap she had clamped on her head.

"You stayed in a box last night? On the street?"

"Nah, not on the street. It's in an alley, kind of," she said matter-of-factly. "Nice and dry. I just didn't know about the nails."

This couldn't be! People don't live in boxes in an alley in the middle of winter. Not in this day and age!

"Look," I offered, "why don't I call somebody and see if we can't find you a nice warm place to stay—one of the women's shelters maybe?"

Her eyes darted with fear, and she reached for her coat. "No!" she shrieked. "Don't call nobody. I don't want to go to one of those places. They'll take him away from me. They don't want people like me should have a dog. They'll take him!" She already had one arm in her coat sleeve and became so agitated she couldn't find the other sleeve. The dog, who had been sitting quietly, sensed her terror and tried to jump off the table, but I held him tightly.

"OK, calm down, calm down. I won't call anyone. Let's just get him fixed up. What's his name?" I asked, trying to change the subject and quiet them both.

"Joey. He's my Joey," she answered, carefully laying her coat back on the cart. "You gotta promise me you won't call no one. Not the cops, not no one. They don't like dogs in those places. They'll take him and they'll kill him!" She laid her head against the dog's. "They kill him, they kill me. We're the same."

"Don't worry," I assured her. "Nobody's gonna kill anyone. Now, what's your name?"

"Lorraine," she answered, pulling her cap off to reveal dirty brown hair as matted as the dog's.

"Lorraine what?"

"Just Lorraine," she insisted.

"OK, Lorraine. I'm going to give Joey a little local anesthetic and sew up this cut."

I anesthetized the area around the wound and neatly sutured

it, following the stitches with an antibiotic shot to prevent infection. While I had the dog on the table, I palpated his abdomen, listened to his heart and lungs and checked his teeth and ears. Considering the life he was leading, Joey was in pretty good shape.

"Has he had his shots?" I asked, knowing the answer.

"He ain't had nothin'. We never been to a doctor," Lorraine told me, not without some pride.

I quickly administered the full complement of distemper and rabies shots, while she watched me warily.

"OK, pal, that should do it for you," I told Joey, ruffled his head and set him down on the floor. There was a terrible paradox about treating this dog. Here I was giving him all the protection modern veterinary medicine could offer, then he and his mistress would leave the hospital to return to the nineteenth-century life of Dickensian street beggars. We're sending shuttles to outer space and Lorraine and Joey would go back to their box in an alley.

I wrote my name across an ASPCA card and handed it to her. "Come back next week and ask for me. I'll take his stitches out."

She put her coat on, pulled the damp wool cap down over her ears and knelt beside the dog to tie the still-wet piece of red blanket around his back.

The snow, which had turned to sleet, pelted against the window in unrelenting sheets, making it impossible to see the East Side Drive and the river beyond. The dismalness of the day was mirrored by the dreadful condition of Lorraine and her dog. Now that I had treated him, how could I send them both back to the cold futility of the streets? The answer was apparent: I couldn't—at least not yet.

There were so many questions I would've liked to ask. Who was she? Somebody's wife? Somebody's mother? Somebody's daughter? Who had once loved her, and did she ever love anybody? What awful thing had happened that reduced her to this rotten existence?

I looked at her face. She was surprisingly young—maybe thirty-five or forty. It was hard to tell. Her skin was leathery from exposure, and the dirt and grime obscured her features, except for the dark brown eyes that alternately betrayed her fear and despair. But what was the use. My questions would serve only to satisfy idle curiosity. There was little I could do to help her further.

She tied the rope attached to Joey's worn collar to her cart and prepared to leave. "Wait, don't go!" I called. "Has he had anything to eat? Have you?"

"Yesterday, we ate yesterday," she mumbled. "We'll get something."

"Wait here a minute," I instructed her. "I'll be right back."

I ran down the hall to the supply closet and loaded my arms with cans of dog food and an equal number of plastic-wrapped packages of dried food, all donated by a dog-food manufacturer. I picked up a bowl and a can opener and returned to the treatment room.

"Here," I said, emptying the contents of a can into the bowl and setting it on the floor. "This is for Joey now." I dumped the other food and the can opener into one of her shopping bags. "And this is for later." I found a tin, filled it with water and put it on the floor next to the already empty bowl. The dog lapped at it gratefully.

His needs cared for, I reached behind the door into my coat pocket and pulled out the tuna salad sandwich I had made and carefully wrapped early in the morning. "This is for you," I told Lorraine. She had been eyeing the dog's food hungrily, and I knew at some point she'd share the other cans with Joey. But for now, this was the best I could do. "Take it in the waiting room. You can eat it there and stay until the snow lets up. At least it's warm."

She took the sandwich. The look in her eyes was more one of surprise than gratitude. "You're a nice man," she said, bringing the tuna up under her nose to savor its pungent smell. Then she reached down and rummaged around in the bottom of one of her shopping bags, finally coming up with what she had sought—a half-empty bottle of Lanvin's men's cologne. "It smells real good," she said, setting it down on the exam table. "That's for you. You're a nice man," she repeated. I didn't want to think how or where she'd gotten it. That really didn't matter. It was her way of saying thank you, and I accepted it.

This time she allowed me to help her push the cart. With the dog tied to it, I escorted her out to the still-empty waiting room and seated her in the far corner, at the end of a row of brightly colored plastic chairs. I fetched another cup of hot coffee from the machine and put it on the windowsill next to her. "Stay here as long as you like," I told her. "No one will bother you."

It was almost eight o'clock. The clinic was coming alive with the arrival of staff and early clients. Unlike the Animal Medical Center, the ASPCA hospital isn't a twenty-four hour operation. Patients are seen only from eight in the morning until eight at night, though there's a clinic aide to tend to the animals and a security guard on duty all night.

Martha Rodriguez, the clinic supervisor, bustled into my treatment room without having taken time to remove her quilted down coat. Martha was chubby to begin with, the coat made her seem rotund. "That your client sitting out there?" she asked impatiently.

"Which client?" I feigned innocence.

"The bag lady! She said you told her she could stay there."

"I did."

"Come on, Steve, you know we can't have people sitting around in the waiting room all day. This is an animal shelter, not a people shelter!" Martha was being unusually officious.

"She's not bothering anyone. Let her sit there for a while. Maybe the snow will stop."

"It has stopped. It's raining ice now."

"Well, let her stay for a bit. I told her she could when I treated the dog's leg."

"Yeah, and gave it shots too, I bet. Who's gonna pay for them? Not her, I'm sure. You guys are all alike. You'd give this place away if I didn't watch you."

"I'll pay for the shots, don't worry. Come on, Martha, the poor woman has no place to go. Be a sport, let her stay. What's the matter with you? You're usually the softest touch in town."

She undid the muffler around her neck and opened her coat, tapping her chest lightly. "That's all over. No more Mr. Nice Guy! In case you didn't know it, *Dr.* Kritsick, *we* are having a crunch. No money! We keep giving things for free, this joint's gonna have to close."

"We may have no money, but today we've got space. So tell me, who's it gonna hurt if she sits there? Who?" I was almost belligerent.

Martha looked at me and then down at her fur-topped boots. Her expression softened. There was the hint of her usual warm smile. "Ah, no one, I guess," she said sheepishly. "Let her stay. I suppose it won't be her that shuts us down."

In spite of the weather, that day turned out to be a busy one. It was late afternoon before I had time to peek into the waiting room. By then, Lorraine had gone. She never came back with the dog to have the sutures removed, but I couldn't forget her. Every time I saw a bag lady on the streets, I thought about her and the dog, wondering if they'd made it through another year.

Now, incredibly, here she was. Still covered with the soot and grime of the streets, she had exchanged the army greatcoat for a worn and stained man's raincoat that hung down to her ankles. On her feet were a pair of high basketball sneakers, so tattered and torn her bare toes poked through. She clutched the handle of the cart, which this time, along with her shopping bags overflowing with newspapers and odd articles of clothing, contained a battered portable TV set. And of course, tied to the cart by a brand-new bright-red leather lead, was Joey. Did the TV work, I mused, and if it did, where did she plug it in? And how had she come by the dog's lead? No matter; somehow they both had managed to survive. That in itself was no small triumph.

When she saw me, her face broke into a now toothless grin. In the intervening years, she evidently had lost what few teeth she possessed when we first met. Aside from that, neither she nor the dog looked any worse than they had that miserable day three years ago. If anything, they looked better. At least they weren't on the verge of freezing to death.

"How are you, Lorraine?" I greeted her. She didn't answer. In-

stead, her eyes darted nervously to Carmen, who was watching
our reunion with apparent disapproval.

"Don't worry about Carmen," I assured her. "I told her you
were my friend. Now what's wrong with Joey?" I knelt down to
pet the dog and once again got a strong whiff of Lorraine. She
hadn't improved in the washing department. That unique sour
smell I remembered so well followed her like a permanent dark
cloud. She shook her head and pointed to the treatment booth.
She wouldn't speak until we were alone, away from what she took
to be Carmen's official, threatening gaze.

I closed the door to the booth, untied the lead from the cart
and hoisted Joey onto the exam table. If it was possible, he was
even dirtier than she. I doubted if he'd ever had a bath, and he
was at least five years old. The minute I got him on the table, he
began to scratch, and I knew whatever problem he had was probably complicated by a bad case of fleas.

"OK, Lorraine, now what's the matter with him?"

She eyed the door warily, as if Carmen were about to burst
through it. "Ears!" she whispered hoarsely, so no eavesdropper
might hear. "His ears—real bad!"

Indeed, the insides of both ears were fiery red and crusted with
the dried ooze of infection and accumulated wax. Before I could
medicate them, they would have to be irrigated with Cerusol to
melt the wax in the canals and clean up the outer ear. I instructed
Lorraine to hold the dog while I flushed and swabbed. Joey sto-
ically submitted to my ministrations, interrupting occasionally to
scratch at the fleas, which were probably more annoying to him
than his ears. When I had finished, I squirted the contents of a
small tube of Panalog ointment deep into each canal. Panalog
was aptly named. It was the universal topical remedy of veterinary
medicine. I even had used it once myself, with great success, for a
bad case of athlete's foot.

"I'm gonna give you some of this stuff," I told Lorraine. "Put
it in each ear twice a day, morning and night. Then massage the
ear like this." I showed her how to fold the ear and rub the outside so that the ointment worked its way into all the ridges and
crevices. "Do you think you can do that?"

She nodded distractedly, still staring at the door. "That woman gonna call the cops?" Her voice was edged with fear. "She'll call the cops and they'll take him away from me 'cause I ain't fit!"

"She only works here, Lorraine. I'm in charge, and I promise no one will take him away from you."

"You sure?"

"I'm positive."

She relaxed just a little, petting the dog lovingly. "He saved my life. Three times, he saved my life. Guys come at me at night, he scares 'em off—like this." She growled and grimaced, showing her gums. "No Joey, I'm finished. Like that!" She snapped her fingers.

I thought about what it must be like for a woman living on the streets at night and shuddered. It was hard enough for someone like her to fight the elements, much less the human flotsam and jetsam she had to defend herself against. Without the dog, it probably would have been impossible.

While I had him on the table, I gave him a cursory examination, checking his heart, lungs and teeth, and administered another set of booster vaccinations. I looked at the leg I had sutured that first time. It had healed nicely, and the stitches were gone. Somehow, his owner had removed them herself. Now for the fleas. They were literally jumping off Joey's back. I was certain Lorraine was as infested with them as he was, and though treating them both was undoubtedly a losing battle, it was worth a try.

"He's got a bad case of fleas," I said, parting the hair near his tail to show her.

"Yeah, I know. We always get 'em in summer." It was another fact of her desultory life that she unquestioningly accepted.

"I'm going to give you some powder to put on him and some shampoo. Is there anywhere you can give him a bath?"

She thought for a minute, scratching her head. "Yeah, I can take him to the fountain in Central Park. In the morning real early, no one's there."

"OK," I agreed, "but make sure you dry him thoroughly. You don't want him getting a chill." We were having a spurt of Indian summer, and though the nights were cool, the days were as warm as the middle of August. Still, it was wise to be careful. I stopped myself in mid-thought and chuckled. This dog probably could've survived the rigors of the North Pole with no ill effects, and here I was worrying about bathing him in eighty-degree weather. Better I should've thought what the city fathers would say if they knew the Bethesda Fountain was being used for a flea dip. That was their problem. Mine was Joey.

"Now what about you, Lorraine. Can you get yourself a bath? If you don't, you're gonna give the fleas right back to him."

She shook her head and mumbled something I couldn't quite understand. I could see the idea of the bath disturbed her more than the fleas. She lifted the dog off the table, and when she had set him on the floor and attached his lead to the shopping cart, she looked at me sadly. "I go to the sisters for a bath, they'll take him from me."

I assumed she meant the Sisters of Charity, who ran a women's shelter downtown. "I don't think they will," I assured her. But what did I know? Maybe they would. "Look, wait here for a minute while I get his medicine. Then you can do whatever you want." I could offer her emergency aid, but I couldn't be responsible for the rest of her life.

I opened the sliding door just enough to let myself out of the booth and went into the night pharmacy next door. I found the flea shampoo, the powder, a flea collar, a couple of tubes of Panalog and as many cans of dog food as I could carry and quickly returned to Lorraine. She was agitated and pacing the small room. The dog sat quietly at the side of the cart, following her every move with his eyes.

"Here's the shampoo and flea powder," I told her and put the bottles into one of her shopping bags. "Rub the powder all over him after he's dry; and here's some food I thought you might want." She stopped pacing, took the cans from my arms, placed them in the other shopping bag and covered them so they didn't show.

I took the ointment from my lab-coat pocket and put it in her hand. "Remember, twice a day, or it won't do any good. If he's not better, come and see me again."

I was beginning to itch as I usually did when I treated fleas. I wanted to get them both out of the room—fast. I knelt and put the flea collar around the dog's neck. "Keep this on him," I instructed. "It'll help."

When I opened the sliding door, Lorraine peered out, checking Carmen's whereabouts. Noting the receptionist was busy on the phone, she tugged on the dog's lead and pushed the cart into the corridor. "You're a nice man. We won't bother you no more." They headed for the exit, Lorraine shaking her head and muttering to herself.

When I turned to spray the exam table with antiseptic, I saw the little china figure sitting on the edge. She had left it there for me. It was a monkey, one of the hear-no-evil, see-no-evil, speak-no-evil trio. This one was see-no-evil, but the hand covering the left eye had broken off. Another thank-you resurrected from the bottom of Lorraine's shopping bag. I turned it over in my hand, wondering if I'd ever see her again. That was one of the odd things about this profession I'd chosen and where I now practiced it. My encounters with people in these little booths were often so intense, their hearts and souls bared to me in their relationships with the animals I treated. Then most of them walked out the door, and that was that. It was like a play in which I was a leading character in the first act and rarely got to see the rest of the action. From my point of view, it usually happened offstage. I never knew the end.

It was well after midnight. Artie Roberts, the overnight intern, had signed in, and there were only two people waiting in the reception area. At last, it was time to go home. I went back to my tiny office, retrieved my jacket from the closet, hung up my stethoscope and threw my dirty lab coat in the laundry. One final look at ICU and I would be on my way.

The residents of ICU had little regard for the late hour. The epileptic Chihuahua had recovered sufficiently to greet me with a series of loud yaps, sparking a contagious yowl from Harry, the Lhasa HBC belonging to that beautiful girl—what was her name? Ah, yes, there it was on the dog's chart, Andrea Walker. I had put her card somewhere, probably in the lab coat that just went down the laundry chute. It didn't matter; her phone number was right there on the chart. I made a note of it so I could call her in the morning. Harry looked alert, the bleeding from the mouth had stopped, and now that he was cleaned up, he was little the worse for his run-in with the car. He'd probably be released tomorrow. That would be good news for the divine Mrs. Walker.

Kenny Gilbert's miraculous high-rise cat was resting comfortably in the next cage. His breathing was regular. He too was on the mend. I moved down the line checking the charts until I came to the last cage, upper right. A small Yorkshire terrier, ears perked, looked out at me accusingly. Oh, my God, Angelo Farrentino, the forty-five-cent dog. Mrs. Farrentino would be furious. In the rush tonight, I'd forgotten to call her. It was too late now; she too would hear from me in the morning.

I walked over to the exam table where Penny Soames was bent over the scalded puppy, rubbing ointment on its blistered skin. "How's she doing?" I asked and put my arm around Penny's slender shoulders.

"Barely holding her own," she said grimly, without looking up.

"If she can make it through the night, I think she has a good chance. Keep her under the heat lamps."

"That's where she's been. I just took her out to put on some more cream. Poor little thing just cracks my heart."

The puppy squirmed on the white towel Penny had laid under her. I could see that more hair had fallen out from the burned areas, revealing the scarred skin underneath. She was still in shock, and Penny's care for her tonight would be critical.

"I hate to leave you with her like this. But there's really nothing more I can do. Besides, I'm just about dead on my feet. Artie Roberts has signed in. He'll help you if you need it."

"Artie Roberts," she sneered. "Him help? You've got to be kidding?"

"Aw, come on Penny, he's not so bad."

"He sure ain't so good. Why do they always leave me with the dummies?"

"I don't know, hon," I shrugged. "Maybe they think you'll teach them something." I kissed her lightly on the cheek and left the room, heading for the side exit and home.

Before I had gotten halfway down the hall, Carmen ran up to me, panting and out of breath. "Oh, *Dr.* Kritsick, thank God you're still here. There's a kitten stuck in the elevator shaft!"

"Christ, how'd that happen?"

Carmen ran alongside, trying to explain the circumstances as best she could. But she was so excited, she kept lapsing into Spanish. Even so, by the time we reached the bank of elevators in the reception area, I had a good idea of what had taken place.

The elevators stop running at eleven o'clock. Usually, the doors are closed, but for some reason one door was left open. About twenty minutes before, a man had brought in a kitten he had found on the street. He had no carrier for it, of course, and the frightened kitten jumped out of his arms, looking for refuge somewhere in the reception room. The man went after it, but the little cat managed to squeeze itself through the space between the open elevator door and the shaft. With the luck attributed only to cats, it hadn't fallen. Somehow it had landed on a narrow ledge and moved along it toward the rear of the elevator shaft where it now cowered.

Artie Roberts and the man who had brought the kitten in lay on their bellies on the floor of the elevator. They had removed a panel from the back wall, and through the opening I could make out the terrified kitten huddled on the ledge.

"Our arms are too short; we can't reach it," Artie said when he saw me. He was a little guy as was the middle-aged black man at his side.

"OK, let me give it a try." Visions of my soft bed and the Late Late Show went right down the shaft as I wiggled between the two men on the floor.

The panel opening was about a foot wide and a foot and a half long, too small for anything but a head, or an arm to get through one at a time. First, I poked my head in and spotted the kitten, small, shivering and frozen with fear on the ledge. I judged the distance to be just over four feet from the opening. I reached in, hoping to grab the cat quickly, but my fingers felt only air. The ledge was farther than I thought.

I stood up to take my jacket off, and the Good Samaritan took my place at the opening. "This is what I get for not minding my own business. Should've left the damned cat where it was, would've been better off," I heard him mutter. Then he looked up at me, a stricken expression on his face. "Hey, Doc, hurry! Damned cat's standing up on the ledge!"

I shoved him out of the way and looked through the opening again. Indeed, the kitten had stood up, its back arched in fear, the long hair standing away from its body from neck to tail in a fan effect. One misstep and it would drop to the bottom of the shaft, three floors below.

"OK, kitty, settle down," I whispered soothingly. "Settle down little kitty. I can't get you unless you sit down nice and quiet."

The cat, its eyes the size of quarters, gleaming yellow in the half-light, mewed faintly. I knew if I reached for it now, the kitten would back up and slip, and that would be it—finished! Cats are so damned perverse. Only a cat could've gotten itself into such a fix, a dog would never be so inconsiderate.

"Come on, baby, sit down," I coaxed. "It's getting so late and I'm so tired. Please, I beg of you, sit!"

Artie Roberts and the black man were lined up on either side of me, absolutely still, afraid any movement they made would cause a noise and startle the kitten.

"What's going on?" Artie whispered.

"How long do you think this'll take, Doc? I got to go to work tomorrow," the kitten's savior asked.

"This isn't my idea of fun!" I pulled my head out of the opening and hissed over my shoulder. "I want to get out of here as much as you do. But I can't get at the damned cat until it sits down. So just cool it for a minute!"

I stuck my head back in the hole. Purring so loudly the sound reverberated through the shaft like a tiny engine, the kitten resumed a crouch. "That's a good kitty," I cajoled. "You just sit there nice and still. Uncle Steve's gonna reach right in and snatch you off that ledge. Nice kitty, good kitty. You stay right where you are—don't move."

Imprinting the kitten's exact position on the ledge in my mind, I brought my head back in the elevator and pushed my arm and shoulder through the opening as far as I could. The metal from the bottom of the panel opening stuck in my ribs and, when I moved slightly, it tore my shirt. I shot my arm out quickly, and the tips of my fingers brushed soft fur. Just another inch and I'd have it. The purring had stopped. Please don't move, little cat, please don't. I pushed myself farther into the shaft. I felt the metal cut my skin, but I reached out and grabbed. "Gotchya!" I yelled triumphantly, as my fingers closed over the scruff of the kitten's neck and I brought the yowling, squirming ball of fur through the opening.

"Hey, Steve, terrific!" Artie Roberts patted me on the back. "If you hadn't been here, we would've had to call the fire department. That's one lucky little cat." He ruffled the kitten's head as it clawed its way up my chest.

"You're bleeding, Doc. Look at that. You hurt yourself?" The black man pointed to my torn short and the ring of blood around the rent. I looked down and assured myself it wasn't serious. Then, feeling like Gary Cooper in the western I had probably missed on TV tonight, I said, "It's nothing, just a scratch," and handed him the kitten.

"It ain't mine," he said, handing it back. "I just found it on the street and brought it here where it'd be safe." He stood up. We were all still in the elevator, Artie Roberts, the man, me, the kitten and now Carmen, who had come over from the reception desk to offer her congratulations.

"What do you mean, it isn't yours? Aren't you gonna keep it after all this?" I was tired, annoyed and more than a little put out.

"Man, I would if I could, but I can't," he said, running his hand through his close-cropped, curly salt-and-pepper hair. "I live in one of those apartments where they don't allow pets. Like I said, I was just doing a good deed. Found it on the street and brought it in here." He carefully brushed the dirt from the elevator floor off his trousers. "Now that I know the cat's OK, I'll be going. You take good care of that little bugger, it's been through a lot!" He gave us a kind of salute and was gone.

"Well, so much for that," I said wearily. "Another drop-off." The kitten now rested inside my shirt, purring happily against my chest. I pulled it out, held it up with one hand and examined its underparts. "First of all," I announced, "*it* is a she."

"I figured," Carmen said. "She's gonna grow up to be real pretty." She chucked the kitten under its whiskers.

"You want her?" I asked hopefully.

"You kiddin', Dr. Kritsick? I already got three cats. Another one, my boyfriend'll kill me."

The kitten was indeed pretty. Just about three months old, she was black with distinctive white markings. White boots on her front paws, a flash of white on her chest and the end of her tail and, best of all, a perfectly round white patch over her left eye that made her look as if she were wearing a monocle. There was something very special about this cat. I didn't believe as the Chinese did that because I had saved her life I was responsible for it. Nevertheless, I wanted to see her well set up. She needed someone who would appreciate the whimsy of her looks as well as compensate with love and care for her erratic beginnings.

Then it hit me, like one of those cartoons where the light bulb goes off over the guy's head. That doesn't happen to me often, but this time it did. Of course, I had the perfect home for her. Fate had sent her to me with everything but a sign hanging around her neck, and I almost didn't get the message.

I unhooked her tiny, sharp claws from my shirt and handed her to Artie. "Will you do me a favor?" I asked.

"Sure, Steve, anything," he answered quickly. Artie was a good egg and not a bad vet. I didn't know why Penny lit into him so badly.

"I'm just too damned tired to walk back to ICU again. Would you take the kitten back to Penny Soames? Tell her to put my name on her. I just thought of a home for her."

"Hey, that's great. She's a cute cat. Do you want me to give her shots or anything?"

"No, I'll come in tomorrow during the day and take care of the shots myself. Just see that she's fed and ask Penny to keep an eye on her tonight." I rubbed the kitten's head one last time. "You get a good night's sleep, kiddo, so you can be charming. Soon, we're gonna put on our selling shoes!"

Chapter 13

Tonight I would see Kate Gilchrist. At last there would be more than just idle conversation in the intensive care ward, or passing at a trot in the corridor, each carrying a sick animal. No, this would be a real sit-down-face-to-face-with-time-to-spare *date*. I had planned it for days—drinks, dinner, the works. I even bought a new suit for the occasion. Nothing was too much. This was the girl who might change my life.

I ran along the park's river path with her name dancing in my head. Ever since she had agreed to see me outside the hospital as a payoff for taking care of her snake patient, I had thought of little else. In fact, I found myself obsessing about her like a teenage boy, oblivious to the sights and sounds around me. My pace quickened. I was running much faster than I usually did. Not certain if my heart was pounding because of Kate fantasies or exertion, I slowed down. There was no need to hurry. It was Saturday. No work tonight—the day was mine.

Slightly out of breath, I stopped and leaned against the iron railing that prevented pedestrians from tumbling into the murky Hudson River. The air was sharp and clean, smelling of salt and brine. The lingering warm days of Indian summer had gone. Finally, in this last week of October there was a crisp snap in the wind that blew across the river from New Jersey. It was cold on my face and it quickly dried the rivulets of perspiration that had escaped from under the twisted red bandana I tied around my head as a sweatband. I zipped my warm-up jacket and hunched over the rail, watching pieces of debris pass on the swift current below. I thought how good it was to be alive and, on this day at this moment, to be here.

Riverside Park meanders from 72nd Street to 116th Street, bordered on one side by the jumble of once luxurious limestone mansions and Gothic apartment buildings of Riverside Drive and on the other by the Hudson River. Its acres of greensward and winding paved footpaths provide an almost rural landscape for the residents of New York's Upper West Side.

Because it has neither the midtown convenience nor the cachet of Central Park to the south, it's never crowded, yet on fine days it too takes on the character of a multiracial Brueghel painting. Mothers sun their babies in carriages, kids play stickball and Frisbee. Lovers, heedless of the activity around them, gaze at each other on the grass or kiss in the shelter of the graffiti-covered tunnel entrance to the park. Bag ladies poke at trash cans, then tally the morning's take of discarded objects while resting their bunioned feet on the dilapidated benches. Teenage black and Puerto Rican boys, hefting enormous "ghetto blaster" semiportable radios on their shoulders, vie with each other in a kind of electronic machismo to supply the surrounding area with background rock music. But Riverside has what no other park in the city has—it's got the Hudson River, and because of that, it's my favorite place to run.

I've been coming here for better than four years, ever since I relinquished the questionable charms of Mrs. Mercado's studio in favor of a less convenient but certainly pleasanter one-bedroom apartment on West 76th Street. Every day I run the asphalt path along the Hudson's edge to 116th Street and back again, a distance of exactly five miles. Perfect for a sprint before work to clear my mind and, incidentally, to stay in shape.

I've come to know the river and its denizens well, taking pleasure in the diversity of traffic that makes its way up and down the wide gray-green waterway that separates New York from New Jersey—the barges laden with goods destined for export to Europe, towed by brightly painted toy-boat tugs; the ocean-going yachts and smaller pleasure craft returning to their permanent

moorings and marine community in the 79th Street boat basin;
the occasional canoe or kayak, manned by a single oarsman
straining against the elements and the strong current as if from
another time and another place; and finally, the Circle Line cruis-
ers, hauling their cargoes of tourists upriver to Bear Mountain
and back down around Manhattan Island. I could almost hear
their passengers exclaim, goggle-eyed, about the splendor of the
skyline and the excitement of the city, then cross themselves at
their great fortune—they didn't have to live here! I knew what
they were saying, because five years ago that might've been me.

But now when I looked across to the Hudson's western shore
and saw Jersey, I thought like a bona fide New Yorker—Ah, the
beginning of the *rest* of the country. And why not? I've paid my
dues. I belong.

To be honest, there were moments during my first six months
in the city when I wasn't certain I could or even wanted to belong. I remember Don Schwartz, a surgeon at the A and the only
born and bred New Yorker I knew then, saying to me with unmistakable New York chauvinism, "We're a kind of environmen-
tal mutation. If you can succeed in New York, you can succeed
anywhere in the world. Doesn't matter where you come from in
the first place, or whether you're a plumber, a teacher, an actor, a
salesman or a vet. If you can do it here, you can do it anywhere. If
you can drive a car here, you can drive anywhere. If you can survive here comfortably, you can survive anywhere. We're the
super-breed, different from the rest of the country. That's why
they don't like us. Even our rats and roaches are stronger and
smarter. There isn't a pesticide developed that can do them in.
Same with the people. Hang in there kid! The air'll get to you—
you'll make it!"

I don't think it was the air, nor do I think I've become one of
Don's mutants, a super-rat. But I have managed to do much
more than just survive. In fact, I've flourished. Standing at the
rail on *my* path, in *my* park, by *my* river, thinking about *my* girl
(even if a bit prematurely), I knew how far I'd come.

I had been at the ASPCA for two years when I received the
offer made by the Animal Medical Center: Would I be interested

in coming over as Director of Emergency Services, head of my own department with three interns under me? Would I? It was an offer hard to resist, but still I wasn't certain.

The AMC is at the pinnacle of veterinary establishments in the United States and probably the world. Organized into specialties, very much like the best human teaching hospitals, it's staffed by the country's leading veterinarians and each year attracts the cream of vet-school graduates. A place as an intern or resident at the AMC is considered a prize plum, a credential that can eventually open almost any door in the profession. So the possibility of a post as head of a service was nothing to be taken lightly.

But I enjoyed my work at the A. It was varied and challenging, and the small yet superb staff provided a familial and exciting atmosphere that would be hard to leave.

"You'd be foolish to turn it down," Harley Petersen said, when I told him of the offer. "I say this to you as a friend, not as the director of the competition. God knows, I hate to lose you. But with a year or two at the AMC under your belt, you can go anywhere and name your price, not to mention what you'll learn." Harley sat on the edge of his desk, his arms folded on his chest, his dark eyes intent beneath his black, bushy brows. I respected Harley, as a vet and as a person. There was no pretension about him, no cute angles. What was—was. "They're doing good things over there, and emergency medicine is a coming field. You'll have the staff and equipment to do a great job. I only wish we had the dough to do it here, but I can barely afford to maintain this place as it is. I've just been told there'll be more cutbacks this year. Jesus, Steve, we can't even hire a pathologist, much less a night emergency unit."

Though emergency medicine was practiced at the ASPCA hospital as a matter of course, it was never organized as such. We just took them as they came. Harley had dreamed about a twenty-four-hour trauma unit, much like those recently started at a few human hospitals. But there wasn't even the money to keep the clinic open after eight o'clock at night, so for the foreseeable future, it would remain a dream.

Harley lit another in his steady chain of cigarettes and dragged on it deeply, the smoke curling out of his nose. "You've got to take it if they want you, Steve. It's a terrific opportunity, and I think you're ready for it now. Emergency medicine is when one's bleeding over here, another's seizuring over there, take that one to X-ray, draw blood from this one and put a catheter in that one. On-the-spot decisions, sometimes three or four a minute. Not everyone can handle that, but after two years in this blender, you can. Do it!" he said with a finality that was hard to oppose.

I had come to the attention of R. J. Osbourne, the Director of the Animal Medical Center, in an odd way. For the past several months, I had been making regular weekly appearances on *Romper Room*, a daily children's television program. Each time, I'd bring with me animals available for adoption from the ASPCA shelter and explain another facet of the care and handling of pets to the show's audience. It was a wonderful means of making as many children as possible more aware of animals and their needs. This tangent in my career came about after I had treated Sandy Davis's dog several times. She was the program's producer, and when she asked if I would be willing to do the show, I jumped at the chance. At that time, I had no idea it would become a weekly occurrence, continuing to this day.

One of the board members of the AMC happened to see me while watching *Romper Room* with her grandchild. She immediately called R. J. Osbourne, and two days later, I was lunching with him and Billy Golden, his Director of Personnel. They treated me like a prize quarterback who had just won the Super Bowl.

What Osbourne wanted, I later discovered, was to kill those two proverbial birds with one person. He wanted someone who could handle emergency services at night, then double in brass during the day making sporadic television public-relations appearances on behalf of the AMC. When the board member called him, he quickly investigated my background and decided I was it.

I wasn't certain I liked this aggressive little man who talked more like a football coach out to make a winning team than the director of one of the country's most prestigious veterinary institutions. And Golden, his shadow, didn't strike me any better. They were "company" men, something I had never run into at Angell or the ASPCA. But the Animal Medical Center was a much larger organization, and maybe that was the way it had to be run. At that lunch, I knew instinctively that the people who worked for the AMC and R. J. Osbourne, were simply a means to his end and therefore expendable. The hospital always came first. But I thought I could get used to that. After all, as Harley said, the opportunity was too good to turn down, and even though it meant working nights and turning my life inside out—I accepted.

That was three years ago, and I've never been sorry. As Harley predicted, I learned a great deal, not only about veterinary medicine, but about myself. Because of my odd working hours, I was forced to spend a good deal of time either alone or with other vets at the hospital. Very few girls I met were willing to wait until midnight or later for the pleasure of my company at dinner, and, until Kate joined the staff, the women vets at the AMC were either married, going out with someone else, or looked like hedge posts. So unless it was a nurse who worked the late shift at one of the nearby hospitals or a stewardess arriving on a night plane from Europe, I was out of luck. For some reason, the nurses never worked out and the stewardess resented my inability to drop everything to be with her during an unscheduled three-day layover. "It's not like you're a doctor tending people on their deathbeds," she said, ridiculing what she called my deadly dedication. "They're animals—dogs and cats. Certainly someone could replace you for a night or two." She pushed our brief and tenuous relationship to the point where I had to make a vocal choice, and for me, of course, the choice was obvious. She returned to Paris on her 747, and I went back to watching the Late Late Show on television.

Though my work was gratifying, after a year or so, I found myself yearning for a more normal life-style, envious of friends who could just pick up and go to a movie or theater, or even a simple dinner at eight o'clock on a Wednesday night. As things now stood, I had to make arrangements months in advance not to work Christmas or New Year's Eve.

On the other hand, I did have the days and every other weekend to myself. I was free to run in the park at two in the afternoon or go to a matinee. There, I would see other able-bodied people and wonder what they did for a living. Why weren't they at work? I even developed a theory that the composition of the crowd at an afternoon movie was a pretty good indicator of economic conditions. Particularly if the film wasn't a box-office blockbuster, I felt with certainty that the youngish men and women in the audience weren't playing hooky from a job to come and see it—they were unemployed. It bothered me sometimes that perhaps they thought the same about me. Once, I even considered having a T-shirt made that read, I WORK NIGHTS!

But in the space of two weeks, life had gone from gray-green, the color of the Hudson, to bright yellow and burnt umber. The change was almost miraculous, and I no longer resented working into the small hours of the morning. Now, at least on occasion, Kate Gilchrist worked along with me. And in the past ten days, it seemed finally she was beginning to regard me as more than just a colleague.

It was almost 4:30 when I looked at my watch and realized better than an hour had passed as I daydreamed at the river's edge. The wind had turned cold and the sun, beginning its descent over Jersey, had become a distinct orange ball in the clear fall sky. I trotted down the path back toward 72nd Street through the tunnel that marked the park's entrance. Someone had recently found an irresistible bare spot on the graffiti-scarred walls and scrawled in big black letters, ST. ANTHONY DOES IT BETTER—CALL 580-4772. I wondered if the message was religious or sexual. Hard to tell, but not worth the call.

Knowing I had only an hour to shower and change, I ran the four blocks back to 76th Street and up the stairs of the once elegant limestone mansion that had been converted into ten small apartments. In better days, the house had belonged to Fanny Brice. The second floor front space I now occupied had been her upstairs parlor. But my landlord, with an eye for the dollar, had utilized the room's gracious dimensions and fifteen-foot ceiling height, effectively cutting it in half by constructing a loft at one end and calling it a bedroom. This, in New York parlance, was considered a duplex apartment, and so it was, except I had to crouch after I climbed the wooden staircase to my bed, else I banged my head on the low ceiling. Middle-of-the-night trips to the bathroom downstairs next to the kitchen were to be avoided, since I always forgot about the under-six-foot ceiling, with disastrous results.

I tried to picture the apartment as it used to be in the 1920s when Fanny Brice was starring in the *Ziegfeld Follies* and the West Side was as much *the* place to live as Park Avenue. The large fireplace, with its rococo moldings, was still there (though the flue was plugged up and it didn't work), so were the three long Palladian windows that made a bay overlooking the street. Even the loft couldn't destroy the room's inherent warmth and charm, and I tried to keep it that way by filling it with early–American furniture and prints I picked up cheaply at junk shops and auctions. I was proud of what I had done with the apartment. Though it was no longer elegant, it was comfortable and uniquely mine. I was anxious for Kate to see it so she could know who and what I was outside of the hospital. Our knowledge of each other was truncated at the doors of the AMC. Tonight, I hoped to change that.

I had arranged to pick her up at the hospital. This was her Saturday on. She would be finished at six. I showered and carefully shaved, spending an unusual amount of time staring at my reflection in the mirror wondering if Kate would still find me reasonably attractive. David used to tell me I had no body image, no idea of what I really looked like. I was always astounded to hear someone thought I was handsome or even nice looking. I think that's because I'm so tall and because it seemed to happen all at once. I grew four inches in a year, as if I'd eaten one of Alice's magic mushrooms. For a time, my hands hung out of my sleeves and my trousers were never long enough. In my mind's eye, I saw myself as a gangling giraffelike creature, fit only to pick the leaves off tall trees. It took a while to get used to my new body, and eventually I did. But in moments of stress, I still revert to that old mental image.

I arrived at the hospital exactly at six, nattily attired in my new beige gabardine suit. I had chosen a narrow olive-green knit tie and a short-collared white shirt. Nothing flashy for Dr. Gilchrist. I had a feeling she liked her men preppie looking, and this was as close as I could come to it. Unlike me, preppie men are never extra tall; they're usually medium height and compact like Ryan O'Neal.

Amelia, the receptionist, greeted me from behind her high-fronted desk, "Hey, Doctor Steve, you're lookin' good!" she said appreciatively. She rarely saw me in anything but jeans and my old army jacket. "Got a heavy date?"

"I hope so," I laughed and headed up the side staircase to the clinic area.

I found Kate in Booth 5 with a patient. I rapped on the room's large window and made hand signals that I would wait for her in the staff corridor, but she shook her head and motioned me inside. Just to see her made my heart jump. Tall and blond, she looked the way people are supposed to when they're from California, which she was. She was not movie-star pretty; her features were too irregular and interesting for that. Her high cheekbones tapered down to a wide mouth and a strong chin, and when she smiled, that little line appeared across her upper lip, just below her nose. But what made her really special were her eyes—big, round blue ones, shaded by a double row of dark lashes. In contradiction to their color, they were warm and snapped with intelligence. She wore little makeup; there was no need for it. Her skin had a glow, as if through some curious California genetic mutation, she carried the sun with her.

"This is Dr. Kritsick. He's Director of Emergency Services," she explained, introducing me to the well-dressed red-headed woman who stood on the other side of the exam table. "Mrs. Rodgers thought Johann here had ticks, and she's been picking at them all day with eyebrow tweezers." I detected a touch of irony in Kate's husky voice, and I saw why when I looked at the little black and tan dachshund lying passively on his back, his short stubby paws folded neatly to his chest, his long ears flat out on the table, perpendicular to the sides of his head. The ten black mammary nipples, perfectly arranged in two rows from his sharply curved upper ribs to well below his belly, were irritated and bloody.

"I'm so embarrassed," Mrs. Rodgers gushed. "I was rubbing his little peeper like he loves me to do." Her heavy gold bracelets jangled as she demonstrated with her hand. "And I saw this little black thing on his chest and then another and another. We were visiting friends in the country, and I was sure they were ticks. I didn't know boy dogs had titties, I really didn't." Though she was easily fifty, she spoke in a feathery, little-girl whisper. "Do you suppose he'll be all right? I'll just die if I hurt him badly, I just will!" She nervously fingered a small gold sheriff's star on her lapel that said STAR in cutout letters.

Kate continued to work on the dog and avoided looking at me. She pressed her lips together, and the corners of her mouth quivered as she tried to suppress what we both knew would be a hopeless case of the giggles. "I don't think there's any permanent damage. I've used an antiseptic cream to ease his discomfort," she told the woman, somehow managing not to laugh. "I'll give you some of the medication. You can use it on him at home, at least three times a day."

Mrs. Rodgers leaned down and kissed the dog's black belly. "Mama take care of little Johann," she cooed. "Mama's so sorry she hurt her best fella, she'll make it up to him just the way he likes when we get home."

Kate could contain herself no longer. She turned away from Mrs. Rodgers and covered her face. I saw her shoulders begin to shake and I knew she was as helpless as I would be if I didn't leave the booth that second. I slipped out the door, closed it tightly behind me and leaned against the wall, laughing so hard the tears ran down my cheeks. People passing me in the corridor must have thought I'd finally gone over the edge. Unable to speak, I could only point limply in the direction of Kate's booth.

Still hiccupping laughs and wiping my eyes, I had almost recovered when she emerged from the booth about five minutes later. She had only to look at me for it to begin all over again. Clinging to each other for support like drunks to a lamp post, we took turns imitating Mrs. Rodgers. "I didn't know boy dogs had titties!" Kate whined, perfectly capturing her client's addlepated innocence. "How could she not know? She's had the dog for two years."

"She sure knows where his peeper is!" I wheezed.

"Why do they always do that? Peeper, pee-pee, thingy, dingus. Why don't they ever call it by its rightful name? Penis!"

"I don't know. They're embarrassed, I guess."

"Mrs. Rodgers wasn't too embarrassed to tell us what she does to him. *Sex and the Single Dog*—if Johann could write, they'd have a best-seller!" Kate killed herself with that one and had to hold her ribs to catch her breath. "Oh God! I can't stand it another minute. Let's get out of here!"

She already had peeled one arm out of her lab coat, and I helped her with the other. The dress she wore under it was a muted blue and burgundy plaid of the sheerest wool. It was gathered in soft folds at the waist and held by a wide crushed-suede belt the same blue as her dress. The tailored collar was open, and around her neck was a thin gold chain from which hung a small gold coin that lay in the hollow at her throat.

I felt an immediate sense of proprietary pride in how she dressed and what she was. It was all of a piece. We looked good together, I thought smugly, and then a year's worth of living flashed through my mind like a mini-movie or a series of beer commercials. We were being ushered to our seats in the theater, skiing in Vermont, lying in front of a blazing fireplace, opening small but important Christmas presents, toasting each other with champagne on New Year's Eve, watching the trees come into leaf in Riverside Park, walking hand in hand on some sunny beach, and finally, we were in the loft of my apartment on a rainy Sunday morning.

"Where're we having dinner?" She interrupted my filmic flashes and brought me sharply back to the present. She had collected her purse from a locked drawer in the cardiology clinic and slipped into the light camel's hair coat she took from a hanger behind the door.

"I've booked a table at the Café des Artistes for eight thirty," I

told her. It was one of my favorite restaurants, warm and glowing
with old-world charm and atmosphere. The food, though slightly
expensive, was excellent. I gave no thought to the price; tonight
was special, and it had been a long while since I had treated myself or anyone else to a really good meal. "I thought we'd have
drinks at Tavern-on-the-Green first. It's a nice night, and we can
walk from there."

She looked at me, and her eyes connected so intently with
mine, I felt the color rise above my collar and something jump in
the pit of my stomach. I wondered if she had any idea of my tele-
scoped fantasies, or that what stood before her now had suddenly
metamorphosed from a grown man to a gangling, moonstruck
boy. Had she glimpsed that poor helpless wretch? It happened so
quickly, perhaps she hadn't noticed.

"That's terrific. I've lived here for a year and always wanted to
go both places but somehow never have." She took my hand in
hers and pressed it gently. Could it be, miraculously, she felt the
same thing? We were headed down the corridor to the reception
area when she stopped and turned to me. "I'm very glad you
made me keep my promise about dinner tonight." She smiled,
and the little line appeared above her upper lip. "I have an awful
way of running from what I really want."

I put my arm around her shoulder and pulled her close. Not
this time, I thought to myself—definitely not this time.

We never stopped talking, and by the time we had finished
drinks and walked the two blocks, hand in hand, from Tavern-
on-the-Green, across Central Park West to the restaurant, I felt
there had never been a time when I didn't know her.

The food was wonderful—I think. It's hard to remember what
we ate, or if I ate at all. It didn't matter, I was so filled with her.
There seemed to be a golden aura around our table separating us
from the other diners. Perhaps it was the double intensity of the
candlelight reflected in her eyes, or the wine we had with dinner,
but I don't recall anyone else being in the restaurant. Yet I know
every table was occupied.

We laughed a lot and told each other about our families, where
we'd grown up, our childhood hopes and dreams and, surpris-

ingly, very little about work or the AMC. When the waiter wheeled the dessert cart next to our table, I couldn't turn away long enough to make a selection. By then, I was hopelessly, irrevocably in love.

I wanted to know everything about Kate Gilchrist, to jump inside her mind and heart, and for a while, she allowed me to do just that. In her low, slightly cracked voice, she told me of growing up in Monterey, California. Her parents had left her with her grandmother when she was two, embarking on a round-the-world cruise on a yacht her father had purchased with a small inheritance. When they returned two years later, they divorced, and Kate's mother snatched her away from her grandmother, who had provided the only love and security she'd known in her young life. Soon after, her mother remarried and moved to Hawaii with her second husband. Kate was evidently an inconvenience in the new marriage, so she was once again left. Her grandmother had died, and so she was shunted to her father and a succession of his wives in Monterey.

Her big eyes filled with tears as she told me the story. I looked at her across the table, picturing her as a child. She must have been extraordinarily beautiful, a blond cherub. It was inconceivable to me that any parent could voluntarily leave a child like that for two years. I thought about my own tightly knit family, and of my mother, who wouldn't leave us even for a weekend when we were small. I wanted to reach across the table and grab Kate Gilchrist to me, making up in one moment for all the hurts she had suffered.

"Oh, it wasn't so bad." With her napkin, she wiped away a tear that had trickled down her cheek. "I had all the material things a child could want. My father saw to it I had a fine education. I was just lonely, I guess. I remember countless hours when I was eight or nine, just sitting under a tree all by myself. I didn't have many friends. But then, of course, I got my horse."

"You had your own horse?"

"Yup," she said proudly, "Loco was his name. He was part quarter horse, part Arabian. I got him when I was ten and I trained him myself. He could do everything but talk. Loco became my best friend. It was because of him I decided to be a vet."

When she talked about the horse, her face took on a childlike quality, so much younger than her twenty-eight years. I found myself staring at her without saying anything.

"What's the matter? Do I look funny?" She wrinkled her nose and squinted.

"No, not at all. I was just thinking. You may sound like Margaret Sullavan, but you know what you look like?"

"What?"

I studied her blond hair, made blonder by the soft candlelight, and noted her incredible round blue eyes. "You look like a large cherub."

She threw her head back and laughed. "Steve Kritsick, that's some compliment! I've been told I look like a lot of things, but never that."

"You'd prefer maybe a Lorelei?" I said with a mock German accent.

"Anything but a large cherub. All I can picture is this five-foot, eight-inch, 126-pound baby bouncing about in a diaper." She laughed again and took my hand. "But I know how sweetly you meant it."

We sat staring at each other sappily until we both knew we couldn't sit there another second longer. I called for the check and made the waiter stand by the table until I had paid it.

There was no question but that we would go to my apartment—Kate lived in a high-rise building on the East Side. But it wasn't just the convenience. "I want to see where you live so I can picture you in the right context when we talk on the phone," she said as we got into a taxi. It would've taken too long to walk the eight blocks to my place.

"I'll show you my early–American furniture."

"Is that better than your etchings?" She twirled a make-believe mustache.

I had hoped to bring her back with me and had left a light on in the living room. The apartment looked warm and inviting. She threw her coat over a rocking chair I had just found and planned to restore and walked around the room fingering everything as if she were committing it to memory. "Oh, Steve, it's lovely. You've made a real home. My apartment has a bed and a couch and some prints I've never hung. I keep meaning to do something with it, but I never seem to find the time. Maybe I will now," her voice trailed off.

I stood behind her with my arms around her neck. "Maybe you will. I'll help." I turned her around and pulled her close against me. Her body was slender and firm. "If everything turns lousy in the vet business, I can always be an interior decorator," I whispered in her ear.

"I hardly think so, Doctor Kritsick, I hardly think so," she said hoarsely, as I led her up the stairs to the loft.

"Watch your head, the ceiling's low," I told her.

"I don't plan to be standing," she murmured.

The sound of rain pelting against the long windows awakened me Sunday morning—just like in my fantasy. I raised myself on one arm and watched her sleep, her blond hair tangled on the pillow like a halo around her head. How lovely she was, and how lucky I was to be on this earth during her time. Once she allowed it, our connection was so immediate that it occurred to me that perhaps we'd known each other in another life. I wasn't into reincarnation or religion, but it was a very pleasant thought that I could take even further. What if after this life we were to meet again and again. We'd always be in different bodies, but we'd recognize each other at once, no matter the disguise.

I leaned over and kissed her lightly on the cheek. She stirred, traced my face with her fingers and turned toward me, continuing to sleep against my side. I wanted to spend the rest of my life with this girl, I was certain of that. I had only considered marrying once before, someone I had met while working at George Carney's. But she had ideas of a life much grander than a veterinarian could offer, so our relationship abruptly terminated. David had said to me at the time, "You got out the dolly dishes too soon. You should've given it a minute and really gotten to know her." He was right. But this was different. I did know Kate. I was sure of it.

I wanted my parents to meet her. Not just to validate my feelings, but to share my pride in her with them. However, they were in Lexington, and barring opening the windows and shouting her name through the rain on 76th Street, there was no one in New York I could bring her to, no one who meant that much to me. No one—except Mrs. Benson.

What a terrific idea! I had told Kate all about her—what an extraordinary woman she was, how close I felt to her and how devastating it was for both of us when I had to put her cat to sleep. I even had shown Kate the kitten I had rescued from the elevator shaft and planned to give Mrs. Benson as a surprise. What better time than today? Now I'd have two surprises for her. I lay back in bed, content with my plan. Kate awakened, and I drew her nearer to me.

Later that afternoon, after a huge brunch—orange juice, French toast smothered in maple syrup and bacon—that we prepared jointly in my two-by-four kitchen, I called Mrs. Benson to make certain she'd be at home. I said nothing to her about the kitten, but I did tell her I was bringing someone I wanted her to meet. "A girl?" she asked intuitively.

"A very special girl," I said, promising to be there in about an hour.

Finding a taxi when it rains in New York is a near impossibility, even on a Sunday. As the first raindrop hits the street, they all disappear underground, or flash their OFF DUTY signs, taking great delight in hitting the nearest puddle and splashing you as they speed by. Our sense of accomplishment was so great when we finally flagged a large Checker cab, we decided to keep him waiting while Kate went up to her apartment to change her clothes. Though it was only three blocks from the AMC, it was raining too hard to walk. "I'll be quick," she said and ran into the modern, yellow-brick building on East 65th Street. It looked like all the other apartment houses constructed in the city in the last ten years, faceless and drab. As if to contradict its lack of originality, it was called The Van Gogh, after the artist. If he could've seen it, he would've hacked off the other ear.

The driver sat in the front seat, contentedly reading the Sunday *News,* while I watched the meter tick. After a quick discussion about how rotten the weather was, we had nothing further to say to one another. Finally, ten minutes later, Kate emerged from the building wearing a long yellow slicker and a canvas rain hat. I could see she wore jeans underneath.

"Sorry it took so long, I was soaked through. Had to change from the skin out."

"It wasn't long at all," I said, eyeing the meter, which had just hit five dollars.

We drove the few blocks to the AMC, and this time Kate waited in the cab while I raced upstairs to the ward and got the kitten, placing her in a cardboard carrier. On the way out, I grabbed a few cans of cat food, in case Mrs. Benson had none left from her Eloise days.

"I hope I'm doing the right thing," I said as we sped through the nearly empty streets back to the West Side. "She said she didn't want another cat. Maybe I'm being presumptuous?"

Kate had taken the kitten out of the carrier. It climbed up her chest and settled itself behind her neck, tipping her hat over her eyes. "No way." She reached up behind her and scratched the cat's head. "From what you've told me, this kid and Mrs. Benson were made for each other. She's a cat person and a cat person couldn't say no to a kitten with a monocle."

Like many of the buildings on West End Avenue, Mrs. Benson's apartment house had once been elegant. Now the only remnant of its former glory was a wizened little man who functioned as both doorman and elevator operator, his threadbare and shiny, greenish uniform jacket worn over a tieless shirt and a brown sweater with big holes in the front. Though I had seen him many times before, he gave no sign of recognition. Instead, without announcing us first, he motioned us into the building's rickety and scarred wood-paneled elevator and carried us silently to the tenth floor.

The old woman's delight in seeing us was apparent when she opened the door to her small, memento-filled apartment, her arms outstretched, her face wreathed in smiles. I bent my head so she could plant her usual kiss on my cheek and introduced Kate to her as Dr. Kate Gilchrist, taking care to keep the cat carrier well behind my legs, so she wouldn't see it at first.

"So this is your surprise, Steve?" She shook Kate's hand with both of hers. "She must be very important, if you're bringing her round to see me."

"She is." I smiled broadly. "And since you're the only other important woman in my life in New York, I thought you should meet."

"You're right." She winked at Kate. She had planned a proper tea and had dressed for the occasion in a long-sleeved, floor-length, dark green hostess gown, with a stand-up collar that came right to her chin. It was probably of her own design and reminded me of the dress worn by the wicked Queen in Snow White and the Seven Dwarfs. I had explained to Kate that Mrs. Benson had once been a theatrical costume designer and that her clothes were still rather dramatic.

She had gathered our wet raincoats in her arms and was preparing to hang them in the bathroom when she noticed the carrier. The holes poked in the side were a dead giveaway, and if they weren't enough, the kitten began to yowl loudly.

"What's this?" She dropped the coats in a heap on the floor and knelt beside the carrier, opening the flap top slowly, as if she almost didn't want to see what was inside.

"Another surprise." I tried to sound casual. "She kind of had your name on her. I hope you don't mind."

The kitten had pushed her small black face out of the opening, revealing the perfectly round white marking over her right eye. Mrs. Benson reached in and gently pulled the cat out, cradling it in her arms like a baby and touching each of its white-booted black paws. "She's wonderful, Steve. She looks like a Prussian general with a monocle and boots. But you shouldn't have. You know I can't have another animal. I'm too old. What if something happens to me? Who'll take care of her?"

Her long dark dress made her seem very small and vulnerable, though today she wasn't using the cane. I ignored the stab I felt as I once again realized her age and physical condition. "Nothing's going to happen to you, you're indestructible! Not only that, you have two personal vets to look after her. Kate's a feline specialist. If that cat even mews wrong, just call one of us," I reassured her.

Carla Benson sighed and sat on the chintz-covered couch, stroking the kitten in her lap. "I'll keep her on only one condition; if anything happens to me, you or Kate must take her. Promise?"

"I promise," I told her, catching Kate's eye.

"Of course we will," she echoed. "But nothing's going to happen to you."

Another cat couldn't have been completely out of Mrs. Benson's mind. Within minutes, she had pulled out Eloise's old litter box and scattered her toys on the floor for the kitten to play with. Her face broke into a satisfied maternal grin as she watched the cat acclimate itself to its new home, inspecting the nooks, crannies, exits and entrances in the small apartment and finally, rolling itself in a ball at her feet.

"Well, I guess I've got myself a cat. Now that she's here I'm really very pleased, though I'm sure she's not as literate as Eloise. Did Steve tell you? I used to read to Eloise all the time. She loved it," she told Kate.

"But that's the wonderful thing about cats, they're all different. It's as if each one speaks another language." Kate scooped the kitten off the floor and sat next to Mrs. Benson on the couch, holding the little cat out at arm's length for inspection. "This one's got such a funny face, she's bound to have the personality to go with it. But she's got to have a name. What're you gonna call her?"

"I knew the minute I saw her. Let me show you." Mrs. Benson got up and crossed the room to a wall of framed photographs. She took one off its hook and brought it for us to see. "Do you recognize her? You two are both so young, you probably don't."

"Of course we do, it's Marlene Dietrich," Kate exclaimed.

"You forget, we watch the Late Show." I held the black-and-white photograph of Dietrich wearing white tie, tails and a top hat. In her right eye was a monocle. The picture was autographed, "To Carla and Will, auf Wiedersehen—Marlene."

"Well, what do you think?"

"Perfect. Marlene it is!" Kate laughed. "Did you know her?"

"*Do*, my darling, she's still alive. Feeble I'm told, but alive. I'll get our tea and tell you all about it."

The table in front of the couch was set with a Wedgwood tea service. Mrs. Benson didn't often have guests, but when she did, she liked to make it a ceremony. While she was in the kitchen, Kate took my hand. "I'm pleased you brought me, Steve. She's delightful, exactly as you described her. Does she really know all those people in the photographs?"

"Every one. Go and look at them, they're all autographed."

Kate was inspecting the pictures on the wall when Mrs. Benson returned with the teapot. "Most of them I *did* know," she said to her. "There are very few left I *do* know. That's the worst part of living to be old—all your friends die before you."

We stayed with her for better than two hours, while she regaled us with stories of her famous friends and life in the theater. She and Kate hit it off exactly as I knew they would, and when Mrs. Benson discovered Kate was from Monterey, that sealed the friendship.

"Monterey, Carmel, Point Lobos—the most beautiful part of the world. Before my husband died, we had planned to move there. How lucky you are to have grown up in such a gorgeous place. Now when I see you, I'll be reminded of all that beauty."

When she had fetched our coats from the bathroom where they had dried, she took Kate's face between her hands and kissed her on both cheeks. "I'm so pleased Steve has found you," she said. "I'm very fond of him, you know. He's what I would've wanted my own son to be." Then she poked me in the ribs. "Now don't you be a stranger. You brought me Marlene, now the least you can do is look in on us every once in a while."

"I will," I promised.

"And bring her with you. A pretty face brightens this room."

"Now that I've met you, there's not a chance I'd let him come without me," Kate said, smiling.

It had stopped raining, and we walked a few blocks before I put Kate in a cab to her apartment. She was on duty at the hospital at

eight the next morning and wanted to spend the night at home. I
hated to let her go, but I understood, and after kissing her long
and well, I hailed a taxi.

"It's been a wonderful weekend, Steve, the best I've had in
years," she said through the rolled down window of the cab.

"See what a good time you can have if you just let yourself?" I
kissed her on the nose. "See you tomorrow and the day after that
and the day after that and the day after that." The taxi drove off,
and I waved it away, literally dancing down the street, happier
than I could ever remember being.

We did see each other almost every night and weekends for
about two months. I'd meet her after work at my apartment or
hers, and the nights we both worked, we'd go home together. We
talked about getting married, or I should say I talked about it. But
Kate thought things were fine as they were, so I no longer
brought it up.

Just before Christmas, I noticed a marked change in her that
was most disturbing. In the midst of what I thought were our
happiest moments, her eyes would take on a sad, faraway look, as
if a transparent shield had dropped between us. No matter how I
tried, I couldn't break through. It was a kind of depression that I
knew had little relationship to the present and for which, I kept
telling myself, I wasn't responsible.

"How can you be depressed?" I would ask her, trying to jolly
her out of it. "You're young, you're beautiful, you love your work
and you've got me!"

"I don't know, Steve. I just don't know," she'd say. "It has
nothing to do with you. Try to understand that. The only way I
can describe it is—I feel as if air is rushing through me, as if I
don't exist."

We were to go to Vermont to ski over the long New Year's
weekend. I had juggled schedules and made deals to switch work
hours with residents and staff doctors, trading July 4th for New
Year's Eve so that we could have time off together. I had planned
to stop in Lexington on the way north to introduce Kate to my
family. The day before we were to leave, I found this note in my
mailbox at the hospital.

Dear Steve,

I've decided to go back to California. By the time you read this, I will have left. I've resigned my position here (I said there were urgent family matters that would take several months to attend to. Please don't make a liar of me). I know I can find a good job without too much trouble. The past few months have been wonderful—the best I've known—but I can't control those awful moods and they're getting worse. If we stayed together, I know I'd make you even more unhappy, and finally, you'd want to leave me. I couldn't bear that. Perhaps someday, when I become a whole person (only what you deserve), we can try again. I do love you.

K.

My hands shook while I read the note. The pain I felt was later replaced by anger and then pain again. For several months I searched for her as best I could, making a nuisance of myself on the telephone with the California Veterinary Medical Association and then methodically calling every Gilchrist listed in phone directories from San Francisco to San Diego, all to no avail. In this day of supersonic transportation and mass communications, she had effectively managed to disappear. I could only hope that someday, somewhere, we would meet again. Maybe by then she'd see herself as I saw her—beautiful, brilliant and loving—a remarkable human being.

Chapter 14

The anticipation I'd felt for the approaching Christmas holidays turned to dread. I had canceled the trip to Vermont; without Kate, it was pointless. Even if I'd found a last-minute companion, the truth was, I just didn't want to go. Perhaps I was dipping my toes in self-pity. The time of year made it difficult not to, since both merchants and media conspired through song and television commercials to make togetherness a compulsory uniform. I had been part of a loving, wondrous *we*. Now I was alone, and each time I heard "Have Yourself a Merry Little Christmas," blaring through every radio and loudspeaker as if New York disc jockeys had no other record in their repertoires, I was a bit more naked.

Word of Kate's abrupt departure had spread quickly through the AMC, and my friends tiptoed around her name, careful not to mention it in front of me as if she had died. Well, she hadn't died, she'd left. And even though on a conscious, intelligent level I knew her reasons for going had to do with things other than our relationship, in my heart was the certainty she'd left *me!* Somehow, I had to pick up the pieces of my life and put it together again without her. Eventually, the physical pain had to leave. The hole in my middle would knit, the awful emptiness would disappear and I would once more find interest in other people and most important—my work.

But now it all seemed impossible. Nights at the hospital were longer and more wearing than ever, though the usual holiday crush of new kittens, puppies and accident cases gave me little time to feel really sorry for myself. I again rearranged the schedule so I would work Christmas and New Year's Eves, much to the delight of the surprised and grateful residents I relieved of duty. There was no sense taking the time now. Who could tell? Life might be better in July.

"Come on, Stevo, you gotta come to the party!" Kenny Gilbert flagged me in the staff corridor, his arms laden with giant bags of popcorn and potato chips. "It'll be going long after you knock off work. What're you gonna do, go home and stare at your antiques? Everyone will be there, even Osbourne. After all, you helped me save the cat that paid for it. The least you can do is show up!"

"I'll try," I said to placate him, though the last thing I wanted was to go to that party. Kenny's long, striped muffler was trailing from his shoulder to the floor. I picked it up and wound it around his neck so he wouldn't trip on it. "Depends what time I get through. Right now, there's a mob in the waiting room."

"Don't they know it's Christmas Eve?"

"Maybe they think we're giving presents with every exam."

"Half-off tonight in honor of Baby Jesus," Kenny laughed. "I gotta get home and make the bed before my guests arrive. See ya later, OK?"

"I'll try, I really will."

"Be there!" he ordered. "Be good for your soul."

"Since when're you interested in my soul?"

"I'm not. I just want you to stop moping." He scuttled down the hall and turned before he reached the door. "Hey, Stevo!" he called. "Merry Christmas!"

"Yeah, Merry Christmas," I muttered, unable to muster much spirit.

Because of the holiday, we were working short staffed, and to make matters slightly worse, Jim Hartley was on duty with me. Though he'd improved some in the past two months, speed and grace under pressure were still not his strong suit. As usual, he was picking and choosing the easy cases lined up on the clipboards next to the night pharmacy door, leaving what he considered the more complicated ones for me. That was probably all to the good, since the one thing he was capable of without supervision was giving inoculations to new kittens and puppies.

I picked up the next clipboard in line, a rabbit imaginatively called Peter, and summoned the owner from the reception area. "Mr. Gould!" I called. "Mr. Harrison Gould!"

An attractive-looking, silver-haired man of about fifty, wearing black tie and carrying a closed wicker basket on his arm, rushed from the reception area. At his side was a little girl of about seven, her face tear stained, her enormous brown eyes brimming with fresh replacements. I led them into a booth, and the man put the basket on the exam table and opened the lid to reveal a white rabbit well on its way to being the size of a prize pig. It sat so motionless in the basket, for a moment I thought it was a large stuffed toy.

"Daddy stepped on him and broke him," the little girl wailed, tears splashing down her small face.

"I didn't do it on purpose, honey," Mr. Gould said quickly, more to me than his daughter, and helped me lift the rabbit out onto the table. "I was dressing for this party we're having," he explained, "and the damned rabbit followed me into the closet. He's always underfoot. But believe it or not, big as he is, I didn't see him. I stepped on his hind leg. I think it may be broken. I'm really sorry."

"Let's have a look." The rabbit was hunkered down on the table, his long ears flat back against his head. I lifted his hindquarters and flexed the right leg. He jumped and emitted a loud, odd sound, not quite like a squeal.

"You killed him!" the little girl sobbed and hurled herself against her father, burying her head in his side.

"No, I didn't kill him," I tried to assure her. "He's going to be fine. Let me show you." I held the rabbit up so she could see he was indeed robust and intact, and with the exception of the leg, which was certainly fractured, in excellent condition. "We're gonna X-ray his leg and put a cast on it. Then he can go home and be with you for Christmas."

She peeked at me from her burrow in her father's jacket. wiping her runny nose with the back of her hand. "He's not gonna be dead?"

"Not a chance. He'll be up and hopping around in a day or two," I promised.

"How long will it take to do all that?" Mr. Gould asked. He took a monogrammed handkerchief from an inside pocket and gave it to the little girl. "Use this, Amanda. Don't use your hand."

"About an hour," I told him. "We're a little backed up in the treatment room. If you want, you can leave him overnight and pick him up tomorrow."

"That would be great. I ran out on my wife and forty guests. I've got to get back." He straightened his black bow tie and tried to rub the residue from his daughter's runny nose from his dinner jacket. "Come on, Amanda. We'll leave Peter with the Doctor so he can be fixed up and we'll get him in the morning."

"No!" Amanda shrieked, so loudly the rabbit's long ears stood up straight. "I'm not going without Peter. I'm not!" Her head was barely above table height, but her short stubby legs stiffened and she planted her feet firmly on the floor and grabbed for the injured animal.

"You don't want to do that," I said, quickly snatching the rabbit off the table before she could grasp him. "He's got a broken leg. You could hurt him if you picked him up the wrong way, and that would be awful, wouldn't it?"

Amanda ignored me and held on to the edge of the steel table with both hands, screaming as her father tried to pull her away. "I'll never see Peter again. He's going where the sleeping dogs go," she sobbed pitifully.

"We had a little poodle, had to be put to sleep," he explained. "The reason I brought her with me was so she'd see Peter was all right. But I guess it didn't work out that way."

"Mr. Gould, hold on to the rabbit a minute." I exchanged places with him and knelt in front of the little girl, bringing her chin around so she could look right into my eyes. "Amanda, Peter is going to be fine. Only his leg is broken, and we have to put it in a cast. That takes time, so he'll stay here with me tonight. He'll have lots of company. There're dogs and cats and even some guinea pigs and a turtle. It'll be like he's at a party. Then tomorrow morning after you've opened your Christmas presents, you can come back and get him."

Some of the hair had escaped from her long blond braids and it hung in fine strands over her ears. Forgetting her father's handkerchief, she wiped her nose again with the back of her hand, her big, teary brown eyes never leaving mine. "You promise he's not going to sleep forever?" she sniffled.

"I promise!" I said firmly. "Besides, Peter's too big and healthy, you must feed him something terrific. He's the biggest white rabbit I've ever seen."

A smile broke through on her stern little face, revealing that two front baby teeth were missing. "Vitamins," she said proudly. "Mommy gives 'em to us both for breakfast. That's why I'm so tall," she giggled, raising her shoulders and covering the gap left by the missing teeth with one hand.

I stood up and tugged her braid. "That's it! I knew it was something special. Well, have his vitamins ready for him tomorrow morning; he'll be home."

Her father sighed with relief. "Thanks, Doctor, I wasn't sure we'd make it through this. Some Christmas Eve. Now, what's it gonna cost me?"

"I'd estimate about $150. That includes his overnight stay, the X rays and the cast. You can pay half now and the rest when he's released or all of it now, as you wish. I'll do the paperwork, and you can pay at the cashier in a few minutes. They'll call your name."

"Peter is a very expensive rabbit," he said, smiling sardonically.

I held the rabbit while the little girl covered his long ears and face with kisses. "You be good Peter," I heard her whisper to him, "and don't go to sleep tonight, not once. You hear?" Then she beckoned me to lean down even further and planted a very wet kiss on my cheek. "Be nice to him," she instructed in a small baby voice that carried just a hint of promise. Amanda was learning fast. She undoubtedly would have a rosy future.

Mr. Gould grasped her hand, anxious to leave. "Thanks again, Doctor, and Merry Christmas."

"Same to you," I said and hailed a clinic aide to take the rabbit to X-ray while I went into the night pharmacy, completed Peter's record and made out the bill. There were still a number of cases waiting to be seen. I would have to get the cast on quickly and get back to them.

Jim Hartley bustled in all atwitter, his limp hair hanging in his eyes, his face damp from perspiration. "Steve, you've got to do something!"

"About what?" I was trying to finish the bill.

"Jonas! He's doing it with some girl on the third-floor stair landing!"

"Doing what?"

"*It!* He's doing *it!* He's screwing her right there on the stairs."

"So what do you want me to do, spank him? He doesn't come on duty tonight till eleven. Maybe it's his Christmas present."

"You're in charge here, Steve, and I don't think it's right for people to be fornicating on the back stairs. If you don't do something, I'm going to report it," he said officiously.

I looked up from the paperwork. Hartley was a self-righteous pasty-faced bastard and he would do just that. If I didn't at least pretend to be as offended as he, he'd report it directly to R. J. Osbourne and then Jonas would be out of a job. He was the best aide we had. I hated to think what working nights would be without him. I wouldn't've traded Jonas for a dozen Hartleys. Some of us had been after Jonas for a long while to finish college and go on to vet school, and he was working at that now. If he got fired, it would be all over.

"OK, Hartley, you're absolutely right!" I feigned outrage. "I'll take care of it as soon as I finish here. By the way, what were you doing on the third-floor landing?"

"I went up to the cafeteria for a Coke."

Little things he did that I would easily accept in other people made me furious. He brought out a streak of violence in me I didn't know existed. Oh, if I could only punch him in the teeth.

Instead, I put my arm around his shoulders in a comradely manner and turned him toward the counter with the clipboards. "See that over there? Ten cases waiting and more to come. There's only you and me to handle them, Hartley, only you and me, and there's no time for refreshment breaks until we've finished with them, understand?" My teeth were clenched and my eyes narrowed. "Now get cracking! I'll take care of Jonas."

I dropped Harrison Gould's bill off at the cashier and went back down the long corridor toward X-ray to get the rabbit. As I passed B-Ward, Jonas stuck his head out of the door. "Psst! Dr. Steve." He motioned me to him. "Did Dr. Hartley tell you?"

"Yes, you idiot. Did you think he wouldn't? Couldn't you find a better place to entertain your friends?"

"I'm workin' tonight and it's Christmas Eve and all. She just came by to say hello. You're not gonna report me, are you?"

"That was some hello! Jesus, Jonas, for a smart guy, sometimes I wonder where you keep your brains. No, I'm not gonna report you, but Hartley might—unless we shove a sock in his mouth. From now on, will you just watch yourself? If you get canned here, your whole future's down the tube!"

Jonas nodded, stuffed his hands in his designer-jeans' pockets and pawed the floor with his high-heeled western boots. I think he might've been blushing, though it was impossible to tell with his shiny, ebony skin. Jonas was tall and reed thin, with fine features and coarse black hair, which lay in closely cropped curls around his head. He was a darker version of Harry Belafonte and, from all the evidence, just as irresistible to women of every age and color.

"OK, enough with the lecture. You know what the score is. I don't have to tell you any more."

"Yeah, I know. But, man, I go to school all day, work all night. Gotta have a little fun sometime."

"Not here, man, unless you want to blow your career. Got it, man?"

"Got it."

"Now, as long as you're here early, how about helping me out with a leg cast? I'm really backed up, and with only Hartley on, I'll be at it till two in the morning."

"Sure," Jonas quickly agreed, "let me get a lab coat."

The treatment room was semibusy. Susan, the surgical nurse, was working on a cat with a bite wound I had treated earlier, and a large boxer lay on another table, restrained by Walter, the other clinic aide. Its stomach had been pumped. The dog had managed somehow to ingest the contents of an entire bottle of Valium. Luckily, his owner found him before going out for the evening, else he'd be dead.

I looked at Peter Rabbit's X ray while Jonas mixed up a batch of plaster of paris. It was a simple fracture, but because of the way rabbits move, a cast would be more effective than a splint. Anesthetized with halothane gas, the big white rabbit lay on his side in a happy stupor while I fashioned the cast around his hind leg with warm, wet plaster. Just as I gave it a final artistic fillip, my beeper went off. "DR. KRITSICK, EMERGENCY RECEPTION. DR. KRITSICK PUL-EAZE" SQUAWK! SQUAWK!

Both Jonas and I had plaster of paris up to our wrists and I couldn't turn off the beeper. I ran to Susan and had her push the little button to shut it up. "As soon as this stuff hardens," I told Jonas, "find him a spot in intensive care. I'll look at him later."

I washed the white plaster off my hands with warm water and raced out of the treatment room and down the corridor to the reception area, a jumble of unhappy thoughts flashing through my mind that rabbits and drugged dogs couldn't blot out. I was tired. Tired of living an upside-down life, tired of working nights and holidays, tired of spending any time at all with the likes of Jim Hartley. I felt alone and generally separated from the celebrating world of parties and presents, and worst of all, I missed Kate desperately. SEASON'S GREETINGS HOLIDAY CHEER, a string of shiny red and green letters announced across the reception-room walls. Some holiday cheer.

"What's the problem?" I asked Carmen at the reception desk.

"Cat—looks real bad." She shook her head, already writing the death notice. "I put them all in Booth 3." She handed me the clipboard with the cat's record.

There was barely room for me to enter the booth. What seemed like a small mob was crowded in a tight circle around the exam table. They were the Riveras, all eight of them—mother, father, four daughters, a son and a tiny baby of indeterminate sex, whom Mrs. Rivera carried in her arms. The entire family was short and fat, the living embodiment of a Botero painting. The children, ranging in age from the baby to the oldest, a daughter of about eleven, were miniature rotund knockoffs of their parents.

When I walked in, the circle parted, and I saw a closed cardboard carton with holes punched in the sides resting on the table. Mr. Rivera opened the top to reveal Misha, a badly emaciated and very sick, orange and white cat.

"How long has he been like this?" I asked.

"Just like dis, yesterday and today," said Mrs. Rivera.

"For about a month maybe, he not been good," Mr. Rivera added. "He kick the water with his foot. He won't drink none."

"Has he been sneezing at all?"

"No. No sneezing, throwing up alla the time." Mr. Rivera demonstrated, cupping his hand under his mouth.

"Saliva, just saliva," his wife said. "Alla the time he look for food, but he can't eat. Today, I open two cans of salmon—like we eat—and he can't."

"He never been mated. Six years old and never mated," Mr. Rivera mourned.

"But he eats a little, maybe," Mrs. Rivera jumped in.

They both began to talk quickly, each contradicting the symptom the other described. I had difficulty understanding, though a quick look at the cat told me there wasn't much left to know.

"One at a time," I told them, "so I can hear. Now, he's eaten a little bit yesterday, but nothing today, right?"

"Right. In six years he never been sick," said Mrs. Rivera.

"And he never been mated. Six years and he never been mated," her husband persisted.

The children gathered around the box as I lifted the cat out.

With what little strength he had, he hissed and spit at me, but not before I felt the mass in his abdomen and noted the difficulty with which the cat breathed.

"And you say he was fine until two days ago?"

"Well," Mrs. Rivera admitted, "last week he have a little swelling here." She shifted the baby to point to her ample stomach. "And yesterday, I notice he not jumping on the record player we have. That's his favorite place. I give him alla the food he like—grapefruit, Nine-Alive, Figaro, but he no want. You think maybe he gonna die?"

I put the cat back in the box, where he lay motionless, mucus matter dripping from his nose. The children, none of whom had spoken, gathered behind their parents in a small phalanx.

"Look, I can't determine exactly what's wrong with him now, but I do know he's very sick," I told them. "He's dehydrated, and there's a mass, probably a tumor, in his abdomen. There may be one in his chest too. He's very uncomfortable and he's having trouble breathing." They all shook their heads and nodded in unison as I spoke. "I have to tell you honestly, the chances of our helping him aren't good, and if we try, it'll involve a fairly big expense."

"How much?" Mr. Rivera asked, fingering his small black mustache.

"If I take him in the hospital and we do a complete workup—blood tests and X rays—the bill will be somewhere in the neighborhood of $250, and that's a bare minimum."

"Aye, aye, aye, aye." Mrs. Rivera was stunned. "You kidding, Doctor?"

"No, that would be it. And for all that money, I can't even guarantee we can do anything for Misha. He's lost a lot of weight, his muscles have kind of disappeared—what we call atrophied—and that kind of weight loss in his case is probably due to cancer."

The very mention of the word cancer caused Mrs. Rivera to inhale with a deep, rasping sound. "You think maybe we should put him away?" she whispered, hoping the children wouldn't hear.

"I think it would be best for you and for him, I really do."

Mr. Rivera thought for a moment. As sick as the cat was, putting it to sleep was a difficult decision for them to make. "You know, it's Christmas an' for the kids I don' wanna do it. But $250 is a lotta money, more than we got now. And if Misha not gonna get better, what's the use?" He looked at his wife for confirmation and she nodded.

The oldest girl began to sniffle, burying her head in her mother's broad back. The other children joined her in a chorus of loud sobs, waking the baby in Mrs. Rivera's arms, who squirmed and let go with an ear-piercing wail. Soon the tiny booth was awash in tears.

Mr. Rivera looked at me helplessly. "You do this so the kids don' see, OK, Doctor?"

"Absolutely," I assured him. "But first you have to sign this release." I handed him the standard form and a pen.

"Listen, Doctor—" he said after he had scratched his name on the release. "Lemme ask you man to man, you think maybe because he never mated, he get sick?"

For a man with six children, I suppose Mr. Rivera's obsession with his cat's lack of a sex life wasn't unusual. "No," I told him, "I'm sure it had nothing to do with it."

When I picked up the box to carry the unfortunate cat out of the booth, the sobs from Mrs. Rivera's corner of the room became full-blown hysterics. I motioned Mr. Rivera to follow me into the corridor. An idea had suddenly occurred to me. "How would you like a new kitten?" I asked him. A little gray part Persian had been found wandering in the reception room last week. It had been abandoned, and we were looking for a home for it.

"Well, I don' know," he hesitated. "It's a boy?" I saw his eyes light up just a little.

"Yes, but he's already been neutered and had his shots. Won't cost you a cent. What do you say? Be a nice Christmas present for your kids."

"Well, I don' know—" He was almost sold, I could tell. "It's healthy?"

"Very. Why don't you let me bring it out so you can see for

yourself?" I knew once the children caught sight of it, we'd have a deal.

Mr. Rivera went into the booth to quiet his distraught family, while I hurried to the prep room and attended to poor Misha. Putting him out of his misery was the kindest thing I could do, since I was certain his illness was terminal. On the way back, I stopped in B-Ward and plucked the little gray ball of fur from his cage.

In my absence, the small Riveras' hysterics had become quiet, hiccupping sniffles, except for the baby, who continued to scream. I had the kitten nestled inside my lab coat, and when I pulled it out and put it on the exam table, the sniffles stopped completely, replaced by oohs, ahs and smiles. Even the baby, who must've sensed the change in the atmosphere, ceased wailing. The children gathered round the table, petting and stroking the little cat, who should've been frightened by all the sudden attention but instead responded with a loud motorlike purr.

"He's beautiful, Mama. Can we have him?" The oldest girl looked hopefully at her mother, while the other kids jumped up and down shouting, "Please! Please, Mama!"

"Ask your Poppa," Mrs. Rivera said, a smile in her eyes.

They turned to him, all with the same fat little faces, and said in unison, "Please, Poppa?"

"Well, why not? It's Christmas, right?" He was most expansive.

The children turned to the kitten, pushing and shoving to pet it and almost smothering it in the process. Misha, for the moment, was forgotten. Out with the old, in with the new.

I found a box for them to carry the cat and instructed Mrs. Rivera to get a new litter pan and food and water dishes for him, in case Misha had anything contagious I hadn't had time to detect. As they trooped out the door, Mr. Rivera lingered behind. "Thank you, Doctor. You did a good thing. But I wanna ask you one more time." He pulled thoughtfully on his mustache. "You sure he can't have no sex?"

"Positive, Mr. Rivera. It's healthier for him that way."

He shook his head. There was no way he could understand, and I'm sure he thought I was dead wrong. "Poor cat," I heard him mutter to himself, "poor little cat."

Carmen saw the Riveras leave and called me to the reception desk. "Dr. Kritsick, there's a guy here with a collie puppy all covered with glue." She pointed to a bearded young man, who held the pup in his arms, trying vainly to keep it away from his clothes.

"What happened?" I asked him.

"I'm not sure. I went out for a while and when I came back, he was all over glue. I'm a commercial artist, and I've got this great big glue pot sitting on a bottom shelf. He must've knocked it over and then rolled in it. I tried to get the stuff off myself, but I need help. I didn't want to use anything that'd hurt him."

"Aha, not to worry. You've come to the right place. I've got just the man for you. He's an expert in such matters." I turned to Carmen. "Get Dr. Hartley, wherever he is. This case is *his!*" I told her gleefully and sauntered down the corridor to intensive care, a new lightness in my step.

I was surprised to see Penny Soames kneeling next to one of the bottom-row cages in ICU. She was supposed to be off tonight. "What're you doing here? Thought you were going to Kenny's party?"

"Nah, why should I get all dressed up to see the same people I see every day, just to have a free drink? Besides, most of them are cruds anyway. Rather be here with the animals." She stroked the ocelot, lying languidly on its side in the cage.

"What about your family? Don't you spend Christmas with them?"

"There's only my dad, and he's in a nursing home. Been senile for the last two years." She made circles with her finger next to her head. "He doesn't recognize me—wouldn't know me if I came and sat in his lap." She sat cross-legged in front of the cage, and the big cat stretched its forelegs out of the open door, affectionately rubbing its head against her knee. How little I knew Penny. We had worked together for over two years and this was the first time she had ever mentioned her father.

She was an odd little person, almost childlike for her twenty-two years. Solitary and shy, her diffidence was often mistaken for sullenness, especially by some of the interns who had tried unsuccessfully to date her.

"You can forget that one," I overheard Jim Hartley tell a new intern. "She's a little dykelet."

It was a rumor that had spread, without any real foundation, throughout the hospital. And though she might've been mistaken for a rather pretty long-haired boy, whose usual mode of dress was a sweat shirt and painter pants under a lab coat, I don't think she was anything of the kind. Somewhere along the line, she'd been too wounded to deal with anybody of either sex. Her connection to the world was her animals, and she handled them brilliantly. Without her, many of the raw interns with whom she worked the night shift would've been in deep trouble. What was traumatic and upsetting to them was merely routine to Penny. But still, there were those who treated her as some M.D.'s often treat nurses—as an inferior.

Recently, I'd asked her if she wouldn't prefer working days so she'd have a more normal life. I could no longer imagine anyone working nights out of choice.

"Are you kidding?" she'd scoffed. "It's like a zoo here during the day. Besides, I feel really needed at night. You need me, don't you? We're truly one on one, because you've got no backup. At night, there's no cardiology or oncology or surgery. There aren't ten staff doctors and twelve residents and fifteen interns. We have to rely on each other. Right? And when I'm with a particularly dumb intern, I have to rely on myself. It's a challenge. Then too, when I come on at night, it's quieter. I have more time to be with the animals, to talk to them, comfort them. Nah, days wouldn't be any good for me."

Penny put her head down and nuzzled the big cat, her straight dark hair making a curtain around its head. "This old girl's doin' real good."

I looked at the incision on the ocelot's belly. It was healing nicely. Josephine was one of the few exotic big cats who had managed to survive for long as a house pet. Now she was recovering from surgery to remove kidney and bladder stones. She was eighteen years old, and we'd treated her many times. Her teeth had been filed down, and she'd been declawed, practices I didn't approve of. I didn't think ocelots should live in city apartments either. Yet this one was healthy and happy enough, according to our standards, and remarkably, had a much longer life span than if she'd been in her natural habitat. But she was the exception, not the rule.

Owned by a couple who had a house in Greenwich Village, Josephine had been cosseted and cared for with a great deal of expertise. Usually, exotic big cats are purchased or given as gifts because they're adorable cuddly things when they're cubs, or because the fantasy of walking down a Manhattan street with an ocelot on a lead is appealing to someone with a sense of drama and no other sense at all. But cubs grow up and become unmanageable big cats, difficult and dangerous to raise in domestic captivity, not to mention the cruelty inherent in keeping a beautiful living creature so far out of its natural environment.

"Come to think of it, what're you doing here?" Penny gently shoved the ocelot back in the cage and closed the door. "I thought you were taking off for the weekend."

"Things didn't work out. I decided to work."

"Yeah, I heard about Kate leaving. I'm sorry, Steve. She was really nice." Even Penny had gotten the news. I wondered if someone had put up a notice in the elevator. "Some Merry Christmas, huh?" she shook her head. She was tending a noisy macaw that was being treated for lead poisoning. He'd been admitted the day before with seizures after he'd eaten paint chips.

"Hello Darling! *Caw, Caw!* Hello Darling!" he screeched, and pecked at her hand as she changed the soiled paper in the bottom of his cage.

"Quit that, Henry, or I'll let you live in filth!" she warned him.

My white rabbit dozed contentedly in the next cage. The cast on his leg had hardened perfectly, and I admired my handiwork. In the cage beneath him, still dazed but recovering after his encounter with the Valium bottle, was the Boxer. I listened to his heart and lungs and pressed his gum to check its color. "These two guys'll be out of here tomorrow, but keep an eye on them for me, OK?"

"Sure thing, don't I always?" She wiped her hands on her white many-pocketed pants. "Hey, Steve, I almost forgot, I've got a present for you. A real Christmas present. Wait right here!" She placed me by the treatment table in the corner of the room and ran out in such a hurry, her lab coat flapped behind her.

I sat on the table and listened to the portable radio next to the EKG unit emit still another version of "Have Yourself a Merry Little Christmas." It was hard to think when I'd had a worse one. Maybe I'd done my time at the AMC. Maybe I should consider moving on. I'd talked with R. J. Osbourne about working days, but at present there were no openings. I could always go back to Angell. I'd heard through the grapevine they were thinking about setting up an emergency medicine service and I was on the list to head it up. As much as I loved New York, getting back to Boston wouldn't be bad. It was a much easier, more civil place to live, just as Angell Memorial was an easier, more civil place to work. Then again, I could always go back to private practice, maybe even set up my own practice. But I'd need money to do that, a lot of money. It had cost George Carney $100,000 to set up his practice, and that was fifteen years ago. Now, to do anything decent, would cost almost twice as much. From inside my chest came that awful restless feeling. I knew it well, I'd had it before. Only this time, I didn't know quite what to do about it.

Penny came back into the room, dark eyes glowing, her slender face lit with an ear-to-ear grin. In her arms was the little black puppy that had been so severely scalded in the bathtub. The pup had grown considerably since I'd last seen her. Her hair was just beginning to come back, but it was coming in in patches, and the tips of both ears and her nose were scarred a pinkish white. She had a red bandana tied around her neck—the kind I use as a sweatband when I run—and her coal-black eyes were bright and alert. Penny put her down on the floor in front of me.

"When she first came here, her name was something dumb,

like Blacky. But she's been fighting so hard to get well, I thought she deserved something better than that. So I call her Rocky, like Sylvester Stallone."

I remembered the night the pup had been brought in, a breath from death. Aside from the severe burns on her neck and head, the tarsus muscles of her hind legs, which would be equivalent to our ankles, were severely affected. The burns had gone deep into the muscles and tendons. I had told Penny then, if the dog wasn't given a program of physical therapy, the joints could stiffen completely and she wouldn't be able to walk. But even with constant care, I wasn't certain the dog would survive.

"This kid's gonna live, I'm telling you," Penny had said with blind certainty. "And if Sister Kenny could make all those kids with polio walk again, we can do it for one small puppy!"

Working in concert with Angela, a day-shift nurse, Penny had seen to it that each of the dog's hind legs was exercised and manipulated fifty times every time it was picked up. The legs were massaged and the burns creamed. Then she was put in a daily whirlpool bath. The pup's care became an obsession with the two nurses. And after a few weeks, Penny took the dog home with her, keeping it under wraps like a great work of art. Though every so often she would tell me of the dog's progress, I hadn't seen the puppy since that first night.

"Now just watch, Steve. You're not gonna believe it!" Her eyes dancing with excitement, she reached into her lab-coat pocket, pulled out a small, yellow rubber squeak toy shaped like a fish and threw it across the room. "Go get it, Rocky! Go ahead, you can do it," she coaxed. "Go on baby. Show Steve. Go get that fish!"

Rocky stood there for a moment, as if processing what had been asked of her. Then, her hind legs still slightly stiff and wobbly, she bounded across the room and retrieved the fish. Pausing to shake it like prey she pranced back, her red bandana flying like a pennant, and dropped the toy at Penny's feet. I felt the tears well up in my eyes, just as they did when Sylvester Stallone finally raced up the steps of the Philadelphia Museum. The distance across the floor of the ICU may not have been as great as the steps of the Philadelphia Museum, but to Penny and that puppy, it was. I'm just a sucker for great achievement, I guess. Human or animal—it always makes me cry.

"Well, what do ya think?" She grinned and poked my elbow.

"I wouldn't've given you a subway token for that dog's chances. You made a miracle, that's what I think."

"Ah, it wasn't any miracle. I just made up my mind the dog was gonna walk." She picked up the pup and kissed it on its hairless ear. "You did fine, kid, real fine." She said it with pride, somewhere between a mother's and a manager's.

"You sure you won't change your mind about Kenny's party? I'll wait for you if you will."

"Nah, like I said, no point."

I took her face between my hands and kissed her on the cheek. "Thanks, Penny, for the best Christmas present." I ruffled the dog's fuzzy, moth-eaten head.

"Have a good time," she called as I left the room. "And Merry Christmas—from both of us!"

It was almost one in the morning when I finally arrived at Kenny's apartment, exhausted, depressed and fully expecting the party to be over. I came only because I thought it would be easier than explaining why I didn't. To Kenny, tired was never a good enough excuse and depression had no place in his vocabulary. Besides, I liked him, and it seemed important to him that I appear.

His apartment, in a worn gray stone building in the East 70s, was over the Hong Kong Hunan Chinese restaurant. When I opened the door to the white, bathroom-tiled vestibule, the smell of egg roll was overpowering. The tantalizing odor slipped seductively up my nostrils, suddenly reminding me how hungry I was. I rang Kenny's bell, but there was really no need; the inside door to the building, mindless of security, was casually open. I mounted the stairs to the second floor, accompanied by Donna Summer and Barbra Streisand singing "No More Tears (Enough Is Enough)." As Kenny had promised, the party was still in progress—if barely.

"Hey, Stevo, you did come. Glad to see ya!" Kenny greeted me and took my coat and muffler. "Fix yourself a drink and have something to eat. It's all in the kitchen." He threw my coat over the bannister in the outside hall and led me through the dim, candlelit room, carefully threading his way between the standing, sitting and lying bodies occupying the small space. The red neon sign from the Hong Kong Hunan blinked on and off through the window, providing enough light for me to see several couples necking on the low, pillowlike couches that formed an L, comprising the sum total of Kenny's decor. Since there was no bedroom in the apartment, I assumed Kenny slept on one of them.

The strong, sweet scent of pot combined with the egg-roll smell which had followed me up the stairs.

"Wanna toke?" Kenny offered the half-smoked joint he held between his thumb and forefinger.

"Nah, just a good stiff drink and something to eat." I poured myself half a tumbler of Scotch, added just a little water and drained the glass as if it were a Coke. I don't usually drink, but if I was going to stay even for a few minutes, I needed something to wake me up. I flinched as it went down into my empty stomach. But the warm liquid felt good and it tapped into a reserve store of energy, making me feel, for the moment at least, somewhere near alive. Now for the food.

A platter of sadly depleted and tired cold cuts sat on the kitchen table next to browning remnants of potato salad. "What happened to the egg rolls? I thought you were ordering from downstairs?" I asked Kenny, who hovered over me until I had chosen three curling pieces of pastrami and salami and slapped them between two hardening slabs of rye bread. With enough mustard, it wouldn't matter.

"I did. We had egg rolls, the works! But that was hours ago. You should've seen this joint. Wall-to-wall people. Everyone was here, even Osbourne. But he was going on to some shindig a donor was giving. You know him, 'Howsa boy, Kenny? Glad to be here, glad to leave!' " He mimicked the hospital's director perfectly. "But Billy Golden's still here, over on the couch with that nurse from New York Hospital. You know the one, I think you dated her."

I did know her. Nice girl. Too nice for Billy Golden. I wondered what his wife was doing on Christmas Eve, if he was here at one in the morning? Billy, R. J. Osbourne's shadow and spy, was not one of my favorites.

Kenny disappeared into the darkness of the living room to change the record on the phonograph. "Enough Is Enough" had played at least three times since I'd arrived. Enough! I washed the dry sandwich down with another Scotch and immediately felt light-headed. Maybe I should just get good and drunk, I was certainly well on the way. I helped myself to a spoonful of the mouldering potato salad straight from the bowl and looked up to see Jim Hartley lounging against the kitchen doorjamb. Kenny wasn't kidding when he said he'd asked everybody. Hartley had left the AMC about a half hour before me. I never thought to ask where he was going, mostly because I didn't care.

"It was so busy tonight, I never found out if you had a chance to set Jonas straight." He brushed his lank hair out of his eyes and adjusted his eyeglasses. He was aching to hear I had.

"For Christ's sake, Hartley, don't you ever let up? It's Christmas Eve. What are you, a monitor?"

"No, but I think something should be done about it, and if you haven't said anything, Billy Golden's here. I'll talk to him."

I felt the rage well up in my throat and I knew my eyes had gone black. Kate told me they did when I got really angry, and I'd had just enough Scotch to let it out. Hartley was the perfect target.

I grabbed him by his tie and pulled him into the kitchen, shoving him up against the wall. "Listen, you self-righteous creep, I told you I'd take care of it and I did. If I hear you talked to Billy Golden about anything—anything at all—I promise next time you're on my service, I'll make your life a living hell. You can bank on it, ya hear?" I pushed him harder against the wall, and he squirmed to get away from me. "You're not gonna make brownie points on the back of that poor bastard, not if I can help it!"

"Let me go, Kritsick!" he yelled. "You can't talk to me like that!"

"I'll talk to you any way I want. What're you gonna do? Tell Golden on me too? Ah, go on, get out of my sight." I released my grip and he slunk into the other room.

Kenny had heard the commotion and came into the kitchen. "What's going on?"

"Nothing new. It's Hartley again. Why the hell'd you ask *him?*"

"Felt sorry for him, I guess," Kenny shrugged. "What happened this time?"

I told him about Jonas and Hartley's threat to speak with Billy Golden. Kenny's big blue eyes widened and his curly yellow hair seemed to stand further on end. "I think it's too late," he said quietly. "Hartley was talking to Billy for about fifteen minutes before the nurse came."

"Ah, shit!" It was all I could think to say.

"Do you suppose he told him?"

"How do I know? But it's probably a good bet." Another wave of fatigue washed over me. I needed air. I needed to get out of there, get home to my bed and pull the covers over my head. The party was in its last stage. I didn't think anyone would miss me, since most of them didn't even know I was there. Kenny walked me to the door and handed me my coat from the top of the pile on the bannister. "Get some sleep. I'll call you if I find out anything, OK?"

"OK. Thanks for the drinks."

"Don't mention it. Remember, you paid for half." I was almost down the stairs when he called over the railing, "Hey, Stevo—Merry Christmas!"

"Yeah, sure. Merry Christmas."

I had walked to Fifth Avenue, halfway across town, before I realized how cold I was. The temperature had suddenly plummeted and it smelled like snow, though none was predicted. The weather bureau was rarely right about snow. Most of the time they didn't tell you about it until it was actually falling. I always thought what was needed for accurate weather forecasting was a window, an arthritic and someone with a good nose. Normally, I would've been excited at the prospect. I was like a kid about snow. The sight of the first few flakes, indicating it might be heavy, brought back the old and wonderful feelings of school being closed, belly whopping on the Lexington Hills and laughing, always laughing. But tonight, I didn't care what it did. I was an adult, a tired, depressed adult. I found a cab at the corner of 72nd and Fifth and took it across the park to my apartment. Ten minutes later I was in bed, asleep.

My beeper went off. "DR. KRITSICK, EMERGENCY! DR. KRITSICK, EMERGENCY! DR. KRITSICK—" I pushed the button, but the beeping wouldn't stop. Then I realized it wasn't my beeper at all, it was the phone. I tried to pick it up, but my arm, all pins and needles, flopped helplessly against the night table like a dead fish. It knocked the receiver off the hook, making it fall to the floor with a head-splitting clatter.

I flipped myself over and managed to grab the receiver with the other hand. "Hello," I croaked groggily.

At first, I didn't recognize the voice on the other end, but then in a sleepy flash, I did, just before she said, "Steve? This is Emily Addison."

It had been more than seven years since I'd last seen her. I was interning at Angell, partly due to her recommendation, when she flew in from San Diego in her own army-surplus P-47 for a testimonial dinner given for the retirement of a longtime Angell staff member. We'd had little chance to talk, but the day after the dinner, she took me for a flying tour of Lexington and Concord, doing loops and barrel rolls over the neat geometric squares of Massachusetts farmland. For those few hours, it was like the old days, only my palms weren't sweaty and my heart didn't pound when I was near her. Emily was no longer the center of my life. By then, I had found new windows to the world. After a short stay, she returned to San Diego. I heard from her sporadically, mostly through cards at Christmas and my birthday, which she never forgot.

She sounded the same, terse and direct. She told me she was

on her way to Boston and had stopped in New York especially to see me. Because of the weather, she'd flown on TWA. "Not as young and reckless as I used to be," she admitted. I looked out the window and saw my nose had been right; it was snowing heavily. She was staying at the Hilton. I gave her directions and suggested she get a cab and come to my apartment for breakfast. "Brunch," she corrected me. It was almost noon.

Carefully placing the receiver back in its cradle without making any further undue noise, I lay back on the pillows for a moment, thinking about Emily. She had to be in her fifties. I did a mathematical computation in my head of how old she must've been when I first met her, better than sixteen years ago. Then, she was probably thirty-five, maybe even forty. When you're fourteen, everyone over thirty and below fifty is the same. I wondered how she looked now. My mental image of her harked back to the time at Dr. Waters's clinic, and I could picture her with perfect clarity. Oddly enough, I couldn't seem to remember how she had looked when we met at Angell eight years later. Perhaps then I was so full of myself, there was little room for anyone else—even Emily Addison.

But now I realized how anxious I was to see her. She'd been so instrumental in the direction my life had taken, maybe she'd be able to take this indecisive sleepwalker I felt I'd become and once again shove him off on the right course. And if she didn't, no matter. At least I'd be able to talk with her, she'd understand. She always did.

Filled with the re-created remnants of my adolescent feelings about Emily, I leaped out of bed too quickly and banged my already aching head on the ceiling. Having made the expansive offer of brunch, I hoped there was something in the refrigerator besides an old container of milk and a stale egg. When Kate was around, we kept it filled with goodies for weekend breakfasts. But lately I'd reverted to my former bad habits, and the mainstays of my diet were junk food and cookies.

Miraculously, I found an unopened package of bacon and a half-dozen borderline fresh eggs. Cracking one open to make certain they weren't rotten, I sniffed it and found it passable. If the eggs hadn't been OK, I would've had to race over to Zabar's delicatessen on Broadway, probably the only place open on Christmas Day, and with the snow, there wasn't time for that. I peeled off the bacon slices, laid them in the frying pan over a low flame, and measured the coffee and water for the Chemex pot. While the coffee dripped and the bacon slowly cooked, I showered, shaved and dressed in jeans and a comfortable shirt and sweater.

A half hour had passed since Emily phoned. She should arrive any minute. I looked around the living room. After picking up a week's worth of newspapers and junk mail, it was neat enough. I chose a cassette from the stack in the bookcase and put it on the player. It was Vivaldi's *The Four Seasons*, if I recalled correctly, one of Emily's favorites. There! Everything was done. Brunch, though not grand, would be ready when she came. I even had time to take two aspirin for the headache that wouldn't go away. Though I was not prone to hangovers, I had a strong suspicion, that's what it was.

I plopped down on the couch, admired my comfortable room and watched the snow fall softly on 76th Street. It had piled up against the windowsills, making dark shadows against the glass. I loved listening to the sound the tires of passing cars made going over the snow while classical music played. For some reason, I wasn't sure what, the odd counterpoint gave me a warm feeling in the pit of my stomach.

The aroma of fresh coffee filled the apartment. I had just turned the bacon and put the finished pieces in the oven to keep warm when the doorbell rang. Emily was here.

I pushed the outside buzzer and opened the apartment door, leaning over the bannister to welcome her. "It's only one flight," I called and watched her slowly ascend the stairs, bundled in a hooded down parka and high fur boots. The still-unmelted snow on her shoulders and around the rim of her hood made it look as if she'd just come off some arctic expedition.

"Sorry it took me so long," she puffed. "People in New York

certainly aren't polite. I waited ten minutes for a cab in front of
the hotel, and when one finally came, some man ran out and just
got in and drove off. Not even an 'I'm sorry,' or 'by your leave.' "

"He was probably a tourist, someone from out of town. New
Yorkers don't do that," I laughed.

"Hmmph!" She pushed back the hood, and I saw that her auburn hair, still piled in a heap on top of her head, had grayed considerably (Emily never would think to have a touch-up), and the
skin around her pale blue eyes had crinkled and weathered. She
seemed slighter, more fragile and delicate than I remembered,
but other than that, the same.

I was so pleased she was here, I needed to throw my arms
around her and hug her, wet clothes and all. There was an uncomfortable split second, when she, in her still-reserved manner
as if to avoid close contact, stuck her hand out to shake mine. But
I ignored it and grabbed her to me. The snow from her parka
stuck to my sweater, turning to water. "God, I'm glad to see you,
Emily." I held her out at arm's length, looked at her and then
pulled her to me again, kissing her on the cheek. I could tell she
was embarrassed by my effusive behavior, but I didn't care. I
wanted her to feel what I felt. I wanted those sixteen years to melt
like the snow. I hoped, eventually, they would.

"Here, let me take your things." I helped her out of the wet
parka and threw it over the stairwell bannister to dry. She removed her high fur boots and stood them outside the door.
Without them, she was even smaller. She was smartly dressed,
still with the same flair, in a gray tweed pants suit, under which
she wore a soft French-blue silk shirt. A small silk scarf of the
same blue and gray tones was knotted around her neck, enhanc-
ing the color of her eyes. Fashion had finally caught up with
Emily Addison.

I led her into the living room, and she looked around, carefully.
"What'd you do, raid an old attic up in Lexington?" she said
saltily, eyeing my yet-to-be-restored rocker.

"I knew you'd be here one day and I wanted you to feel at
home." I smiled, but I meant it. "Come sit here." I indicated the

couch, the only really soft piece of furniture in the room. "Would you like a drink? I can rustle up a Bloody Mary real quick."

"No, that's coffee I smell and that's what I want. Hot coffee. I'm cold right down to the bone. Been living in sunny California too long, have to get used to these Eastern winters again."

"Nothing like 'em, right?" I poured a mug of coffee for her and one for myself.

"That's the one thing I can't say I've missed." She smiled, showing her still-white, even teeth and wrapped her hands around the mug to warm them. "Now, tell me about yourself. How you are. What you've been doing."

"First, tell me how you like your eggs so I can get them going. Bacon's all done."

"Sunny-side, if you can do them?"

"Of course I can do them. You taught me, remember?"

"So I did," she said. "So I did." I caught her looking at the room again, taking in every nook and corner, like a cat acclimating itself to new surroundings. She went to the cassette player to turn the Vivaldi over and stopped at the bookcase, noting the other selections. "You've got some nice things here, Steve, very nice."

"You're pleased?" I called from the stove, where I had carefully cracked four eggs into the pan of melted butter.

"Not that it matters, but yes, I am pleased. You turned out all right." I heard the smile in her voice.

If only she knew how much it did matter—how many times I'd bought a record or a tape and thought, Emily liked that, or a print or a rug that was like one she had, or how often I did something at work that reminded me of what she'd said long ago. I realized only recently what an enormous influence this small, iconoclastic woman sitting on the couch in my living room had on my tastes and, of course, on my life. Did it matter? She'd probably never know the extent of it.

The eggs began to sizzle in the pan. The toast popped up from the two-slice toaster, and I buttered it while the white part of the eggs browned slightly around the edges. Perfect! The yolks were intact. I slid two eggs onto each plate, laid four pieces of bacon around them and brought them to the small, round oak table I had set for us next to the nonworking fireplace.

"Brunch is served, madame," I announced with fanfare, pouring more hot coffee into our mugs. The table looked kind of elegant. I had found matching silverware and even used the linen napkins Kate had bought.

"It looks wonderful, and I'm ravenous," she said cutting into the perfect yolk so that the yellow liquid oozed onto the bacon.

We sat at the table for hours. I made more toast and another pot of coffee. We laughed and reminisced about the days at Dr. Waters's and we talked about now, or I should say, I did. I told her about the AMC, about the politics of the place and how wearing and discombobulating it was to work nights. I told her of my restlessness and my indecision and, of course, I told her about Kate. She listened carefully, nodding and occasionally offering an opinion. But somewhere in the middle of it all, I looked at her pale blue eyes across the table, and the expression in them was different than when she first walked up the stairs. Now, they were as I had remembered them, warm and caring, at least for me.

Perhaps what I had seen before was fear—fear that the closeness we'd once shared would no longer be there. I was afraid too, but I chose to ride over it. Emily, being much more reticent and conservative, had to wait to find out. As I knew it would, the snow had melted. A lot had happened in between to both of us, but that unique friendship we'd had before she left Lexington for San Diego still existed. Only one thing was different—I had grown up. Now it was my turn to listen.

She spoke of her practice in San Diego. She had shared it with another woman vet whose lawyer husband had just retired and wanted her to retire too so they could travel. She and Emily decided to sell out to a younger man. "I could've stayed with it, but he was interested in being part of a group practice, and that's not for me. I have my ways. I don't want a bunch of wet-nosed kids telling me how to do things," she grumped. "Besides, I've been in California long enough. Climate's bad for you, fries your brains."

"So what're you gonna do?" I poured her another cup of coffee.

"That's why I'm going up to Boston—actually, the Cape—as soon as the weather clears. I've bought a practice there in Truro."

"Truro?" I knew it well. I'd spent summers there as a kid. "Truro's fine in the summer, but winter's cold as hell and nobody's there then."

"Not true," Emily said matter-of-factly. "There's a sizable year-round population. Winter slacks off a bit, but the summer's so lucrative, what with summer residents and tourists, it's enough to carry the practice all year long. I can kind of knock off in winter. Read, write, maybe travel a bit. Fellow I bought the practice from had it for twenty-five years. Did very well. But now his health isn't good, and he has to be closer to Boston."

"You sure you won't be lonely?" The question was a projection of my own feelings about living on the Cape year round.

"Certainly not." She was emphatic. "I've got the dogs, new ones, of course. The old fellows you knew died a couple of years ago. And if I want, I can always fly anywhere I please, I'll have my plane, one you haven't seen, a bright blue Cessna," she said proudly. "Then too, I'd been thinking—I mean, I wasn't certain of your situation here, but I thought perhaps—" she hesitated.

I thought I knew what she was going to say and teased her along. "Yes, you thought perhaps what?"

"Well, I thought perhaps you might like to come on as my associate. I'd give you a fair share of the business, and I'm not going to live forever, you know. Then it would be yours."

"How do you know I wouldn't be one of those wet-nosed kids, telling you what to do?"

"It would be different with you. My husband used to say, 'Fair exchange is no robbery'; he was right." She smiled gently.

I understood now how important it was to her that we reconnect. That's why she waited until we'd talked for hours before telling me about Truro. She had to be sure what she'd known in the boy was still in the man. Last time we'd met, I might've given her reason to doubt it.

I remembered that summer day so long ago, flying in her plane over Lexington and Concord, when the only thing I wanted in the world was to be with Emily and help her take care of animals. Now that it was no longer a boyish fantasy, I wondered if it was the right decision for me to make. Isn't that always the way? You want something so badly you can taste it, and if you wait long enough, you can have it—and then what?

"Working with you would be wonderful, Emily. You know I've always wanted to do that. But I don't know about private practice now," I said honestly. I told her about the possibility of the emergency medicine service at Angell, though I emphasized it was still only in the rumor stage.

If she was terribly disappointed that I didn't immediately jump at her offer, her face betrayed nothing. She was too rock-ribbed for that. "Working at Angell again as head of your own service would be a fine opportunity, Steve. And as much as I'd like you to be with me, if I thought it was better for your career, I'd recommend you do it." She had been playing with the napkin, twisting and twirling it. Now, she laid it on the table and reached across and took my hand. "Look, you don't have to make any decision today, this minute. I'm not taking over the practice for another two months. Why don't you think about it. The offer's there if you want it." She looked at her watch and stood up abruptly. "My God, it's almost 4:30. I've got to get back to the hotel. I'm expecting a call from Truro."

I got my own coat out of the closet and helped her into her parka, waiting while she stepped into her fur boots. Despite her protestations, I decided to go down into the street with her. Getting a taxi might be difficult.

"I'm not that old," she said huffily. "I can still take care of myself."

"I know you can, Emily. I just wanted to spend a few more minutes with you." Actually, that was true. I felt discomforted by the last part of our conversation as if I had let her down. By walking with her for a bit, I hoped to ease it. But life rarely cooperates, and no sooner had we stepped out into the snow, than an empty cab slowly made its way up 76th Street. I hailed it and handed her up over the mound of snow created by the snowplow that had passed earlier and then into the taxi.

"It's been a terrific afternoon, Emily. I'll think about what you said and call you within the month, I promise."

"That'll be fine, Steve. But promise me something else; promise that whatever decision you make, it won't be just to please me or anyone. It'll be because you really want to do it!" She leaned out the cab door and kissed me on the forehead. "Remember, it's got to be for you, Steve."

I closed the door, and the taxi noisily clanked away on its skid chains, disappearing in the heavy snow. I stood in the snowbank watching it go, until I was suddenly aware water had seeped into my loafers, thoroughly soaking my feet.

The phone was ringing when I got back in the apartment. I answered it while taking off my wet shoes and socks. It was Kenny Gilbert. "You're not on tonight, right?"

"Right."

"Well, I've got some news for you, won't keep until tomorrow. Jonas has been canned."

"When?"

"Today. Hartley did tell Billy Golden last night, and they sacked Jonas this morning. Merry Christmas!"

"Ah, shit! Couldn't the bastards at least have waited?"

"What difference would that make? I thought you'd want to know."

"Yeah, thanks Kenny. Thanks for calling."

I picked up my shoes and put them near the radiator to dry, hoping the toes wouldn't curl. Poor Jonas. It was a dumbass thing to have done, but Hartley was a son of a bitch to have ratted on him like a prissy schoolboy. I'd fix him when he was on my service. Somehow, I'd fix him. But what would that prove? Only that I could play the same game of petty, backbiting politics he did—they all did. More constructive to find Jonas another job. Maybe Harley Petersen could use a bright guy like him at the A. Of course, the reason for Jonas's firing would be on the grapevine by morning. Though I didn't think Harley would pay any attention. He was better than that.

I knew now there were things other than my upside-down life-style indicating I should move on. But where? Emily's offer was certainly a good one, and it would please her so much if I came along with her. Then I remembered what she'd said: "Do it because you really want to do it!"

I went upstairs to the loft. There was a good movie on television, James Stewart in *It's a Wonderful Life.* I'd already seen it twice, but I flipped on the set, lay back on my bed and watched as if I'd never seen it before. I'd make all those decisions—for me, for Emily, for the AMC. I knew, eventually, I would. Only like Scarlett O'Hara—I'd think about them tomorrow.